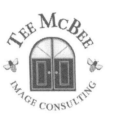

Second Edition

MASTERING
YOUR
EVOLVING
STYLE

30-DAY WARDROBE PLANNING JOURNAL

by TRACI MCBRIDE

Scan the QR code for
a welcome video by Tee

or search:
goo.gl/TFtftW
(case sensitive)

CINCINNATI, OHIO

MASTERING YOUR EVOLVING STYLE
30-Day Wardrobe Planning Journal
2nd Edition

by: Traci McBride
Tee McBee Image Consulting

Copyright 2018 © by Traci McBride

ISBN: 978-1-947553-93-4

Imprints.com

Publisher:
SE Imprints, Cincinnati, Ohio
(513) 464-9782
SEImprints.com
Sales@SEImprints.com

Printed in the U.S.A.

Table of Contents

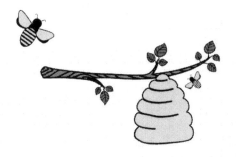

Download a free PDF

Tee's top 10 Tips to Freshen Your Look

Scan QR code or google:
https://goo.gl/TUeauh

Dedication and Acknowledgments

A lifetime of experiences has led me to write this book. I can't count the number of people who have played a role in bringing me to this spot in my life. Some knowingly, like my sister, friend, and publisher Kym McBride. Others unknowingly, like the cashier at the grocery store, the woman at a garage sale and countless FaceBook and networking acquaintances.

My passion is teaching and guiding others to reveal the best version of themselves—everyday, yes, even on weekends, my friends, helping them to reveal another perspective with which to see themselves. None of us are standing still in our lives; there are so many moving parts to living. This book is dedicated to those who know this and want to evolve their style and wardrobes.

I've learned so much from the women who have invited me into their most intimate place, their closets. The stories and experiences in dressing rooms across the cities where I've shopped are hilarious and numerous enough to fill another book.

It's exciting that you decided to read this book and use it to evolve not only how others see you but how you see your best self.

Thanks for joining me on our journey to a deeper understanding of ourselves.

Filled with Gratitude, *Traci*

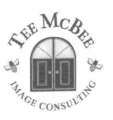

How to Scan QR codes
(funny little box of dots)

QR Codes (Quick Response Codes) are just shortcuts to more information on a product, service or as in our interactive books, to more specific content.

QR codes are the wave of the future. How do we know it's going to be a wave? Apple has just built in a QR reader in your camera app in the latest ISO version. Just hit your camera app, point the camera at a QR code and it will automatically show you the website location, tap it and you will be taken to new content! This is how we can make print books interactive! The wave of the future!

Step one: [If you don't have the updated IPhone] Download a free QR code reader into your smartphone by searching the App Store. In the app store, search "QR Code Reader." There are quite a few to choose from. We would suggest you find a free one such as Quick Scan by iHandy, Inc. It's simple to use. For Android phones, QR Code Reader by TWMobile is free and works well. If you have the latest iPhone IOS 11.0.2 or later, a QR reader is built into the Camera app.

Step two: Once the app is downloaded, familiarize yourself with the operation. If you chose to download the iPhone app by iHandy, Inc. as suggested, all you need to do is tap the app on, and hit the lightning icon that is in the bottom/center of the app. A little box will appear with a green moving scan light and you hover your smartphone camera over the QR code you want to read. The Android app is slightly different; the targeting box appears automatically. If you're reading a QR code on your computer screen, you can scan it too! It works like magic!

Just try to get the QR image into the box. Don't worry if the image isn't sharp; the app will be able to read it. Then it will open up a window that has an open button. Tap it. It will automatically open the webpage with the video/ audio or additional information on the product or service that you wanted to know more about. With the Android app, there may be several options presented after the QR code is recognized by the app; choose "Browse website." Pretty simple.

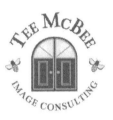

3 Questions you ask every time you go in your closet

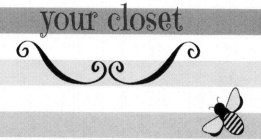

- Who Is Your Audience ?
- What Are You Wanting to Communicate ?
- What is the Weather ?

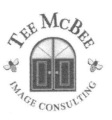

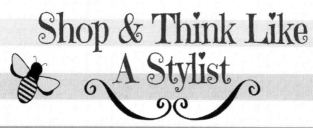

Shop & Think Like A Stylist

Identify Your Style Words

Need **VS** Want

Create A Written Plan

Know Your Closet   (Use Photo Look Book)

Power Colors   (Focus on Palette)

Shape & Cut   (Tailor For Your Body)

Fabric   (Think Care & Wear)

Fit, Fit, Fit   (Plan on tailoring)

Mix-ability   (Create More Looks with Less)

Garment Orphans   (Avoid them)

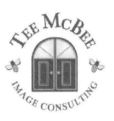

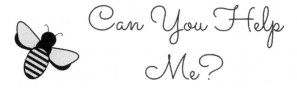

Can You Help Me?

Writing books is a joy. But to get them into the hands of those that need my book is really out of my hands and *squarely in the hands* of my readers.

People read reviews before purchasing so:

Could you please write a review on **Amazon**, **Barnes & Noble**, **GoodReads** or anywhere else you frequent.

It would mean the world to me.
They say if you don't ASK you don't get. :)
Thank you,

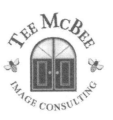

How to use this book

When we know better we do better. When it comes to personal style and wardrobe, I have learned a few things from being in closets with hundreds of women over the last ten years:

- Keeping it simple is the key to being consistent.
- Being objective with yourself will keep you on track.

Break your style down into steps. Anything in life is easier when you work it step by step. You didn't get where you are today overnight; over your life, you have developed habits, beliefs and mindsets that have gotten you right where you are. Some have worked and moved you forward and made you feel good while others have made your life more challenging, leaving you feeling uneasy.

The same key steps work for evolving your personal style. Simple leads to being consistent, and being objective helps you to see things the way they are, and not as you might want them to be.

Several pieces of information will make shopping and dressing as effortless as possible.

Style Words to guide you,
Know your Power Colors so you invest in the right colors.
Use your Body Shape I.D. to invest in the right cuts, proportions and fit for your NOW body.

Use the pages of this 30-day Wardrobe Planning Journal to:
- Coordinate this journal with your *Look Book*; that will help you to choose the appropriate outfit for reaching your goals each day.
- Monitor how you feel in your clothes; this is very powerful as it affects every interaction you have throughout your day.
- Create an on-going workable plan that you can use for shopping as your style evolves. We shed garments as time goes on for a variety of reasons. This process of journaling about dressing can be very informative as you and your lifestyle continue to evolve.
- Create a *system of organization* in your closet; think about how this organization can relieve stress and time.
- Use the journal to assist in planning business trips and vacations with *Effortless Packing©*.

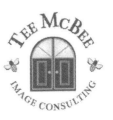

Introduction

I am perfectly imperfect and I embrace that.

I actually love that I can embrace that fact. However, that wasn't always true. Curvy, full-figured women over forty aren't embraced by mainstream media, fashion or retail. Yes, things have improved over the last few years, but if I walked into any women's plus department right now, I would find uninspiring mannequins wearing boring basics for which no one took the time to accessorize with shoes, purses, jewelry or scarves. More often than not, the sales staff will be less than fashionable. Although the collections may have some designer names, they are boring and over-priced. It's like the powers that be don't understand us.

I am often asked how I became a wardrobe stylist / image consultant. It's hard to condense my reply to a short sound bite. I happen to have an old soul and at a very young age was very independent, which was a challenge for my mother. Mom became a widow at twenty-six with three young daughters to raise. I was only two at the time. Family members have told me that I was difficult when it was time to get dressed. I expected my mother to lay out a complete outfit each day for my approval before I would wear it. If I didn't like something about it, or it didn't match, I did not get dressed, no matter the threats, spankings or pinches by my older sisters.

Oh my—the writing was on the wall! By eleven, I was interested in the HOT PANTS trend! Well, I wasn't a tall, slim, little girl like my friends in the neighborhood, I was curvy—what Sears & Roebuck called Husky! Ugh. I watched as my mother tried to force her opinion of what my oldest sister should be wearing. Oh my! The fighting, tears and anger in that dressing room! My middle sister and I hid under the racks of clothes and heard all that frustration.

13

My oldest sister, still traumatized to this day, hates wearing appropriate clothes and would live in her mumu if she could. Many clients have had similar experiences, that's **why I make sure my clients have a good time in the dressing room!**

Fast forward to my early thirties—this is when I lost my mojo. After having my second child and being able to stay home for a few years, I constantly compared myself to skinnier, prettier, hotter moms. I was frumpy, dumpy and hadn't lost the baby weight. While those other moms wore shorts at the baseball field, I wore black and anything to cover up. Since I didn't feel good about myself, I avoided many events. I hated my body and my clothes. I couldn't even talk to people without being completely self-conscious. Obviously, I had some work to do on my self-image! **That's why helping women focus on their best assets has become an ongoing goal of mine.**

As I became an observer of my life more than a participant, I learned about others in the process. I learned to read a person's body language, facial expressions and amped up my listening skills. I started out working as an office temp and then transitioned into a hostess in model homes, where I was able to put what I was observing and learning to use.

Within nine months of being a weekend hostess, (a person that supports the sales representative of customized homes), I was offered a chance to be the sales rep for my own housing development! I said, "No thanks, I don't know enough." My husband said, "WHAT? What do you have to lose? An hourly weekend job?" So I went in the next day and said I'd do it! Looking back, others saw in me what I did not see in myself. Luckily, I just went with what they told me I could do and remarkably it worked! I was very successful working with clients, from selecting their home site, to discussing all the details of building a house, right up to handing them the keys to their new home. My confidence soared. *I now use my enhanced people-observation skills to support my clients by identifying the core issues that are blocking them.*

With five years and a sold-out development behind me, I decided to go to school for my real estate license. Another life lesson: working with a large office of women, *I observed how the way a women dressed directly influenced the type of clients they attracted and the level of success they achieved.*

As the economy began tanking in the mid-2000s, I realized the fabric of the industry was changing into something that I did not love anymore. But what was emerging was my compassion for women. I empathized with their limiting thoughts and daily struggles.

Through my observations of people, and with my highly developed people skill sets, I realized the image component was the key to every success in our lives. If a woman feels good about herself, she can go out confidently and do anything. I turned my focus to image consulting.

My superpowers are the skill of observation, my old soul, my intuition and my ability to see in others what they don't see in themselves. Being objective and seeing one's gifts and strengths doesn't come easily for most women. I give that to my clients; it is what I love about what I am invited to do each day of my life.

My purpose is to help build confidence and influence in others, which is a pretty amazing life purpose!

I have had a very successful local business, but my thoughts recently turned to how can I help more women? I have chosen to write this book to help not just my face-to-face clients in Northeast Ohio, but for all women out there.

Your wardrobe is an expression of who you are at different points in your life. I really feel that your personal presence, enhanced by each and every outfit that you choose to put on your body, is how you share that story. Uncovering your personal style is the greatest gift you can offer yourself. My hope for this book is that it assists you on your journey with your story, and gives you tools to embrace **the perfectly imperfect you.**

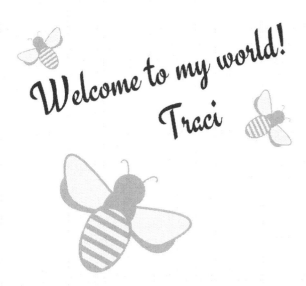

Welcome to my world!
Traci

Step 1:

Determine

Your Personal

STYLE

Words

These are words which you choose, they are the action words you want to express to the world in your life each day.

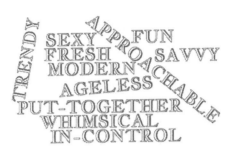

Choose words that describe you or who you want to be. The goal in using these Style Words is to translate those words into your personal style. When you look in the mirror do you feel and see those Style Words? For example, on another day, as you dress for a date, do you see sexy and bold? Is your visual image amplifying that?

Many times, you might feel and portray more than one of your style words and other times, just one. Style words are very powerful when you dress, shop or plan your wardrobe. Style Words can change as you reach different milestones in your life. It is good to check-in with yourself to see if your Style Words need to evolve as your life evolves.

When walking into a store or shopping online there are so many options to choose from that most women become overwhelmed. Many ladies share with me that they are easily influenced by the cover of a catalog, displays in the store or the sales clerk's opinion. Whatever drives your decisions, it is best to take along your personal shopping criteria (body shape, power colors, style words, etc.) to make those choices easier. You need to invest money in your wardrobe as carefully as you invest in stocks and bonds.

Your wardrobe influences your life every single day.

Step 2:

POWER

COLORS

Knowing about Power Colors will be very helpful as you perform your Closet Detox. Building your wardrobe around a palette of colors that enhance, freshen and love you—saves you time, money and energy.

Do you know if your skin undertone is COOL or WARM? Knowing this will save you from being so influenced by the color of the moment or the season. It isn't meant to limit you to a few colors for the rest of your life. It is so you invest your money in colors that play well together and support you getting the right "shade" or hue from all colors. Color is energy. Color influences not only you but those around you that are being influenced by you.

Color influences your facial skin tone. It matters because you want everything you wear near your face to flatter your skin tones and make you look fresh, energized, and balanced. Also, when you invest in garments in your Power Colors, you will see how effortlessly they all go together, giving you more looks with fewer items.

Understanding your skin undertone is key. Typically, you are either a yellow or blue or neutral undertone, this goes for all races. There are methods demonstrated online to support you in figuring out your undertone. (Google search: determining skin undertones) But I believe it is best done by a professional.

Let me share how I do it with a client.

1. Look at the naked face in natural light near a window or out on the deck, not in direct sunlight.

2. Cover your clothes with a white cape and a white cap to cover your hair. Your hair and clothes will alter the appearance of your skin tone, so you want to remove their influence during this exercise. Your hair will change color over your lifetime. If you go from brunette to blonde or red or purple obviously that will impact your best colors, but it will not change your skin tone. Hair color will impact the intensity of your power colors. For example, you may need to modify your palette from a bold teal to a lighter teal. The intensity of the palette changes.

I use a professional system tool, but some image consultants use a draping system that you too can use by using fabric swatches or garments from your closet. (It isn't always easy to see the slight differences; I suggest getting someone to assist you.) Now that you have done #1 and #2, you can drape different fabrics next to your face and see if that color washes you out or enhances your skin tone. As you do this, watch certain areas on your face. Look at the thin skin under your eyes, does it absorb the colors and make you look muddy or grey? How do the colors influence your eyes—are they more vibrant or dull? By this I mean, are the whites of your eyes bright white or dull yellow.

Observe your lips; are they grey, blue or natural pink. Do this multiple times until you see the changes. It takes a bit of time to train your eye to see the undertones so don't give up. During this process, your friend or assistant will need to help you.

Use the mirror. I don't simply tell clients the type of coloring I have determined, I show them so they experience it. When you see how the colors influence your skin, causing you to go from looking ruddy, haggard or splotchy to looking evened out and brighter, you can't help but be motivated to remove all those unflattering colors from your wardrobe! Your power colors will be your secret weapon when adding to your wardrobe.

> *Disclaimer:*
> If you are a heavy smoker, drinker or tan heavily, this will influence how your skin tones appear. Those practices affect your natural vibrancy. Over time, age will make changes to the way your coloring appears. Through his fifties, Paul Newman had eyes that were bright and vibrant, but as he progressed in age, his intense blue eyes dulled down. His skin tone didn't change.
> The brightness or vibrancy changes noticeably for most people as they age.

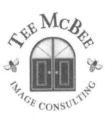

Step 3:

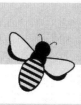

BODY SHAPE I.D.

Identify your Body Shape to invest in the right cuts, proportions and fit for your Now body. Most women identify their shape incorrectly.

Let me break it down for you. Clothing can mask a body shape. The only true way to find your actual shape is to take measurements because the numbers don't lie.

Be sure to measure:
- Outer shoulder
- Bust
- Rib cage
- Natural waist
- Hip

You will be one of the following but possibly share characteristics of two shapes but with one being the more dominant shape. I use these shapes rather than fruit because I believe it gives more clarity.

Example for determining a body shape:

Recently, I measured a client. While she had many curves—a plus size with a full bust, arms and tummy—she does have a natural waist that is 5" smaller than her hips. So, it's not a well-defined or dramatic waist like an hourglass. She is slightly larger in the hips relative to the shoulders.

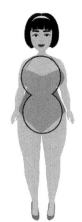

The client measured:
Shoulder: 50"
Bust: 51"
Rib Cage: 45 ½"
Natural Waist: 47"
Hip: 52"

She was a Figure 8.

A Figure 8, as used here, has the top of the eight slightly smaller than the bottom and with some definition at the waist.

BODY *Shape* I.D.

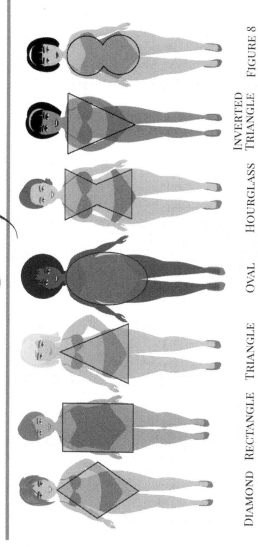

DIAMOND   RECTANGLE   TRIANGLE   OVAL   HOURGLASS   INVERTED TRIANGLE   FIGURE 8

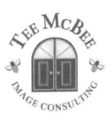

Step 4:

CLOSET DETOX

The Real Estate in your closet is priceless regardless of its size.

I have found most women can make an impact on their own by removing the dated, tired, ill-fitting garments. And before you ask— absolutely, you need to try on each item that you plan on keeping in your closet or drawers. *(Of course, it could really help to ask for help from the professional eye of a stylist.)*

I often hear "I thought I could do it on my own from what I've learned on TV or in magazines." Honestly, many women do a pretty good job putting themselves together—except where they have a blind spot. That blind spot can take a toll on their image and opportunities.

How to Mentally Prepare for a Closet Detox:

Let's talk frankly here. Closet Detoxes have a tendency to bring up a lot of repressed feelings and beliefs. Simply by going through each item, you might hear thoughts in your head that are exposing old unconscious beliefs.

- "Oh, I can't wear brown and blues together, mom told me that when I was a kid."

- "Never mix your horizontal or vertical stripes!"

- "I remember this dress, when mom saw me in it she was upset with the cleavage."

- "I remember my husband really loved me in this!"

- "Last time I wore this, a guy at work asked if I was wearing my daughters outfit; I'm too old for this."

- "I remember I loved this jacket, I got it when I was in New York for my friends 40th birthday, I never wear it; it never really fit very well, but I can't get rid of it."

28

If you listen, you will find a litany of statements or thoughts that rush by as you clear out the items in your closet. But, inside those statements lie hidden beliefs and thoughts that have been influencing what you wear or purchase every day—even if the remark was made two decades before! Why take up this valuable real estate with decade-old beliefs about garments? Ask yourself, *Does this belief service me? Is this my belief or someone else's?* Either way, you can change it.

THE CLOSET DETOX — STEP BY STEP

Just like remodeling any room of your home, it gets worse before it gets better. You need to tear it up before you can put it all back together in a NEW AND IMPROVED way. Right?

Well, that is the same with your closet and wardrobe. February and March are the best time to take inventory and be brutally honest about what is working and honoring your now body and what is not.

You'll need the following:

Boxes, baskets or big trash bags labeled as follows:
- Perfect
- Keep after tailoring
- Sell
- Donate
- Rag Bag

CLOSET DETOX is a very liberating process and great Feng Shui too! Having an organized, uncluttered closet and bedroom will lead to greater ease and flow when you prepare for your day—and better sleep too!

Women don't usually take the time to go through every single item and try it on. But that's how you make the best decisions when you select the box to throw the items into.

Two reasons we never find time to clean out our closets:

- Too much to do. If the task even makes it onto your to-do list it keeps getting pushed to another day.

- Interruptions. The kids need a meal, or a ride. Your commitments and energy are all tapped out.

Think about how much time you spend searching for something in that closet, trying garments on then taking them off again. Some women have shared with me they change three to five times before settling on what to wear each day! Over the year, that is huge time waster that sabotages your self-esteem.

While a first time CLOSET DETOX with me is time consuming (approximately four hours), it will feel like 30 minutes! We stay focused, evaluating each item in front of a mirror, and discussing why each item is a keeper or in one of the other categories mentioned above. No one needs fifty pairs of black pants or shoes or tops. Really! You will fine tune what honors your body and build a flexible wardrobe that takes you to all the occasions of your life, but not a magazine model's life. What is a reasonable number of black pants/shoes/tops? A reasonable number of black pants would be two or three at the most and only if they are different cuts such as a straight cut versus a bootcut.

I usually begin with a bottoms-up approach—pants, skirts, and shorts —especially if you prefer pants to anything else, since so many measurements need to be right for the pants to look their best. I have some clients that experience the most frustration getting the right fit on pants, and others that easily find pants that fit like they were made for them.

Everyone's challenges are different, and we adjust as we go. The woman who easily finds well-fitting pants has an abundance of them, but because her top half might be harder to fit she has fewer tops to go with those pants and vice versa for those who have trouble with well-fitting pants.

Another common situation is this: because a woman can't get a good fit in a garment she is on what I call a *quest* to find the perfect fit, so she buys everything even remotely close to a good fit. All this accomplishes is an abundance of *garment orphans*.

You might find that you need multiple detoxes depending on the combination of emotions and the quantity of clothing you own.

Perhaps you love color and have lots of it in your closet. In your DETOX, first focus on your:

- POWER COLORS. Weed out what does not make you look fresh and energized with an evened-out skin tone.

- Next, focus on your best fit, style, fabric and proportion since you determined your BODY SHAPE I.D. Try on each item from your closet in front of a mirror. *This is where most women begin to justify purchases or have a difficult time being objective. Getting support from an honest friend will be better than doing this on your own.*

This process can be a mess at first (call it controlled chaos), but it is really the only way to evaluate each item. Determinations are to be made; is each ill-fitting item worth tailoring or would you rather purchase something else?

Next up will be the shoes. Avoid building a perfect outfit and ruining it with the wrong shoes. Let go of anything dated, tired, clunky, beat-up, or painful to wear. Some shoes may be worth investing in a professional repair. Knowing how often you are going to reach for a particular shoe or boot is key to knowing where to invest your money.

Many clients have an abundance of scarves they have collected, received or inherited over a lifetime. Many women have shared with me that they don't really know how to incorporate a scarf into their wardrobe, or they aren't sure how to layer prints and multi-colors. Sometimes they just don't like scarves around their neck. If something has sentimental value to you, find another way to honor the memory. Again, this is where your POWER COLOR will come in handy—to help you eliminate or pass along the scarves that just don't fit your new style or color palette. Do you like scarves but aren't sure how to wear them? Google *how to tie a rectangle scarf* and an abundance of Youtube videos will pop up. Choose one or two techniques and practice until you've mastered them.

Next up will be your accessories. Now that you have a handle on your style plus your best neckline from your BODY SHAPE I.D., best proportions and POWER Color, we can make decisions about your jewelry. Of course, your preferences all play into every decision made.

Finally, take a peek at your outerwear. In colder climates, you need a wardrobe of coats. Several different types of casual, wool, leather, professional, evening with a variety of prints, texture and color. Thinking of each season will be the starting point. Different weights from early to late fall then early to late winter, early to late spring as well. This is a wardrobe you build over the years; stick to classics and avoiding *fast fashions* that don't have staying power.

As you go through these steps during your CLOSET DETOX, the goal is to create a shopping list of items to enhance and build upon the garments that made the cut to stay.

By making room and shedding what isn't working, you open a clear path to owning all the items you need. You will own less, but have more complete looks and outfits.

Tee's Tip

Take notes when ideas pop into your head regarding changes in your wardrobe; you will need this information in Step 6 when you create a plan for Power Shopping.

Step 5:

CREATE
A
LOOK BOOK

AND WHY IT MATTERS

This is the secret sauce to your success!

Most women get overwhelmed creating a new look each day as they go. Many times, it is why many women wear only a small portion of their wardrobe and repeat the same look over and over. That will suck your energy and creativity while wasting time. Instead, I recommend blocking out time for self-care by playing with your clothes for an hour or two every season.

Pull out garments you are not currently wearing and partner them with new combinations. Start by hanging or laying them out in good lighting so you can see the colors and details, then mix things up. Once you have some combos you like, put them on to be sure they communicate on your body. If you still love it, snap a photo for your Look Book.

This Look Book can be stored on your smartphone or printed very easily. As you plan your week, referring to your look book will maintain your peace of mind and save the time it takes to change multiple times each day. Many clients ask me to make them a printed look book. They keep it in their closet so they can choose their outfit before bed each night.

Now that I've laid it all out for you step by step, are you ready to plan and commit to yourself, putting hard dates on your calendar to complete the steps?

Here is a link to a video showing how I make a look book for my clients: **goo.gl/teYa4z**

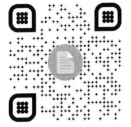

Step 6:

CREATE A PLAN

BEFORE POWER SHOPPING

I have clients who love to shop. Others call me and admit they hate shopping and easily get overwhelmed when they must do it. Now they might like buying gifts for others but finding clothes for themselves is too daunting.

Walking into a store that overflows with a thousand options can be stressful. That is why we use the process of elimination.

SHOP Like a STYLIST every time you shop, this is the key! *(see the checklist in the front of the book)*

Avoid:

- Shopping haphazardly (without your list/Look Book photos)

- Shopping under stress for a last minute event

- Shopping randomly to fill up time or just hanging with friends. You will spend more when others are egging you on to buy things that are just fun and don't have staying power in your wardrobe.

Use your tools to remove most of the options available but that are not in your plan.

- Know your closet and have a digital version of your LOOK BOOK. This will keep you on track. As you shop, focus on what you need for your basics, which you are freshening up or expanding. Know your garment orphans so you can find other pieces that can work with them to create complete outfits.

- Stay within your Power Color palette to cut the store's options in half. The majority of clothes are either warm or cool colors. You are in only one of those categories. Don't even touch anything not in your palette.

- Knowing your Body Shape I.D.—the best cuts, necklines and proportions for your 'now' body shape—will narrow that half down another half.

- Fabric. Always consider the care of an item and choose for the best wear and tear. If you don't want to iron or dry-clean, don't buy it.

- Next, using your Style Words and lifestyle will reduce your options to a manageable size. For example, if your words are *professional* and *conservative* then a brightly colored large print isn't something that should appeal to you. Instead a classically cut blazer in your power color that can partner with the basics back in your closet would be a better choice.

- Fit Fit Fit! *Budget for tailoring*. Be sure the seams sit on your shoulder bone, not off your shoulder. Always button items even if you won't always wear it that way; you want to be sure it fits you properly. The most common tailor tweaks are in the bust area of jackets and blazers, sleeves, waist of pants, hems of skirts and dresses. Factor tailoring into the cost of every item you purchase, it will convert a good fitting garment to a great piece!

- Need vs Want. When shopping for yourself, stay focused on your list of items needed to supplement what you already own and have identified as great fit, style and message.

Tee's Tip

Q: What do you do when there are warm and cool colors in one garment?

A: What color is the most prominent? If it is in your color palette, go for it.

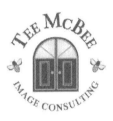

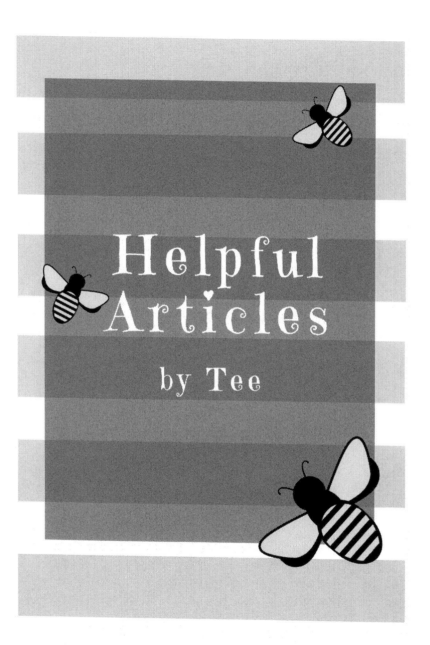

Helpful Articles

by Tee

The Importance of Tailoring 101

Since I spend an abundance of my time in closets all over Northeast Ohio, I many times find suits or dresses that have been abandoned due to some unflattering fit issues. My advice is always to compare the investment in tailoring against the money to purchase something new.

Regardless of shape or size, we need to have a good tailor on speed dial. Whether purchasing any new garment, the key is to keep an eye on the details of the fit. Each woman tends to need the same areas tailored on almost everything.

Example: I have a client that wears a size 14. With certain brands, a 14 is a perfect fit for her length, thigh, seat, and hips, but the waist is usually an inch or two too big. She expects to spend another $15 to tweak each new pair of pants. She has that calculated into her clothing budget.

Example: I have a petite client who is on the shorter side of petites. She is 4 feet 11 inches, so even when shopping in the Petite department, she will need to tailor a majority of her purchases to adjust the length of skirts and dresses. When she finds a top or blouse that is not available in Petites, she weighs the tailoring cost to shorten the garment against the joy the item will give her, as well as the flexibility of the garment as part of multiple outfits. She also needs to evaluate how much detail is involved in the shortening—pleats, buttons, patterns, lining, etc.—as that will determine the cost of tailoring. More detail equals more investment.

Example: Another client is a petite with a short waist, a large bust and narrow shoulders. When she selects tops, blouses, and jackets that fit the largest part of her body, her bust, she often has to tailor the sleeve and the waist. Many times to fit the bust, the shoulder seam sits off her shoulder. If left as is, this will look sloppy and ill fitted. So she must compare the total cost, including tailoring, against the cost per wear value. Reworking a shoulder can be expensive, depending on fabric, lining, pads, and detail. We have found that this year's abundance of ponte knit blazers has been a blessing for her particular fit issues. We have invested in a few of those in her power colors—perfect for pulling a professional look together!

Men have a long history of tailoring their suits, and many stores provide an on-staff tailor for exactly this purpose. Men also have narrow shoulders, wide shoulders, short waists, thick or thin legs, etc., so they have always viewed the tailoring investment as part of the over all cost. Even though they typically spend more on each suit, the cost per wear is low because they wear it on a weekly basis.

Some women think they can avoid tailoring by just rolling back the sleeve or rolling the waist if those areas are too long. I hope you can see the value of paying attention to the details for the details speak volumes about you.

The Most Common Things Women Get Wrong

- Speakers should not wear black against a dark background because they will appear as a floating head, causing a distraction for the audience.
- Typically, in small gatherings of women friends or colleagues, dark seems to be the rule where it should be the exception. Black or dark grays, day after day, homogenizes you. For example, if several women are applying for a job and they are all wearing black or grey, which of them would stand out? What if one of them were wearing some a colorful scarf and shoes with a matching purse, and a broach? You would be drawn to her because she is communicating that she is confident, modern, and detail-oriented. She is willing to take the extra step. If you want to appear as a smart, savvy professional, project that visually. Are you that kind of woman?

Wear Black Deliberately, not as your Default.

I find that when I'm around women who wear black almost exclusively, it drains my energy. It also communicates to others that they are bored, uncreative, or perhaps lazy.

Now don't get offended ... hear me out. I spend a lot of time in closets. Most of the women I work with have numerous pairs of black pants, skirts, and dresses. I help them sort through and decide how to best let go of a majority of these garments.

For example, I have a lovely client who had 39 black pairs of pants! Yes, each was different in some detail, such as the cut, pockets, weight, fabric, trim, etc. As she tried on each pair for me, we chose the ones that best fit her body shape, purpose, and style.

Another woman had every variation of black dresses, 22 in all. We used the same method to narrow them down.
Probably the largest number I've seen in a garment category was black shrugs – 96! Most were slightly different, but many didn't honor her body, either too long, too big, or too similar.

All of these clients purchased these items one at a time. Over time, shopping here and there, they thought each item was completely different from anything they had at home.

I often find the reasoning for owning so much black is a body image issue. They figure they will look slimmer. Usually, it's more about hiding a size or shape that they are not happy about and wanting to just disappear.

Wearing Black Deliberately

As soon as you learn new ways to take the best of your black apparel and energize it with texture, print, layer, and color, your whole wardrobe will expand. You will appear modern, fresh, energized, and outgoing, all while flattering your figure and feeling confident.

Develop a Signature Look to Reach your goals

Think about what you want to visually express. Research proves that 65 percent of all communication is visual. What are your clothes saying about your personal brand? Developing your signature style requires knowing who you are and what you want others to remember about you before you have opened your mouth.

Here are some tips for women and men:

The fit of your clothes will always be number one in my book, regardless of the cost of the item. It is vital to have the clothing tailored to your body, sleeves perfectly hemmed, the break in your trouser just so, and no pulling and tugging at your waist or buttons.

Pay attention to proportion; know your body shape. The cut of each garment should flatter that unique shape. For example, wide hips give you the opportunity to put more emphasis on your upper body. Men can widen the lapels; women can add button detailing on jackets or punch up and visually add width with a scarf.

Know how color interacts with your skin tone, especially near your face. Men should pay attention to the color of their shirts, ties, and pocket squares. Women should do the same with collars, jewelry, and scarves. Know how colors communicate to others:

Red: Action/Angry/Passionate
Purple: Creative/Imaginative
Blue: Trust/Loyalty/Integrity
Green: Balanced/Self-Reliant

Remember the details: polished shoes, leather purse or briefcase, updated and flattering eye wear, watches or jewelry that go with the mood of your outfit. Grooming must be top notch. Watch out for overly aggressive scents. Manners and etiquette often have room for improvement; brush up on yours and avoid pointing out the faux pas of others.

Don't Buy into the Hype

Just because retailers sell it, and push it, and tell you everyone must have this season's trend, don't buy into it. As an image consultant who has spent many hours in women's closets for several years, I often see the aftermath of buying into designer and retailer hype.

Yes, I know it's hard to resist sometimes. It's cute; you see it displayed in clever arrangements in all the stores; the style and fashion TV and print media bury you in smart glossy photos and tell you THIS will make you stylish! Heck, even Clinton Kelly ("What Not to Wear") has admitted that, as an editor for a fashion magazine, he had to suggest that all women should wear red lipstick to be sexy—because the lipstick company was a major advertiser. Now he will tell you that that was a lie; only wear red lipstick if you have a nice mouth and white teeth, as that will be the focus. If red doesn't enhance your skin and mouth, DON'T wear it!

I often find "garment orphans" in closets. Items that women will admit were attempts to look stylish, but it went wrong. Either they were not able to pull a complete outfit together with the item, or each time they put it on, they didn't feel comfortable enough in it to confidently pull it off. Eventually, they took it off, hung it up, and stopped trying it on all together.

All of this investment ends up being wasted. Studies show women have in their closets at any one time $6,000 to $10,000 worth of garments, accessories, shoes, etc, but they only wear $2,000 to $4,000 of it!

Now I'm all for investing in yourself but invest in a wardrobe that flatters your lifestyle, your body shape, your personality, and your skin tone. Your budget will thank you. Your clothes will have a more useful life.

The other common situation is playing it safe and ending up with a sea of black garments with pops of color, which often drains their color, imagination, and creativity. As a result, they look older, bored, stuck and exhausted. Many women only own and wear solid blouses, solid pants, solid jackets and solid shoes. Good Lord, where is the inspiration? Heck, even bankers deserve to show some personality!

No one I know is born with a style manual; thankfully it is a learned talent. Let yourself off the hook. You do not have to be great at everything!

If I need a landscape design, I hire a designer. When I need to do my taxes, I hire a CPA. When I need an electrician, I hire one! The point is knowing when you need help, a little or a lot. Together, you and your stylist can evaluate all the components of your wardrobe. The stylist looks at you with a fresh perspective, considering your shape and proportion while listening to your goals and understanding your day-to-day lifestyle. This will establish your *Signature Style Recipe* and the nuts and bolts of creating it.

So while a *Closet Detox* is the first step, it certainly isn't the only step needed. Your personal brand is an ever-changing journey as we elevate, mature, and develop into the next stage of our lives. The best part is that you can begin at any point and any age.

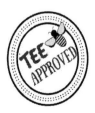

Create a Mood with the Colors you Choose

The calendar says it's spring—and what better time to bring a new dimension and experience to your life than by transforming your closet inside and out with new colors. Invigorate your outdated suits, shirts, and ties while energizing your networking events with one of the new, hot color trends of the season. A fresh blouse or two can instantly change your mood, ambience and energy.

When selecting colors for your wardrobe, it's imperative to know the **Power Colors** for your skin tone and what mood you are trying to achieve, how you intend to communicate, and, more importantly, which colors you really love and feel confident wearing. Color reveals bits and pieces of our personalities. What are you revealing?

For thousands of years China, India, and Egypt have studied the philosophies and relationships between color and energy in order to strike a spiritual balance in their lives. So before you head down to the store, here are some insights into the mood-provoking colors of the rainbow and the energies they emit. Be mindful to always invest wisely and with a plan when it comes to that all important communication tool, your wardrobe.

Red: Dynamic and Bold. Its intensity has a stimulating and exciting effect —a warm and seductive color that exudes power and confidence.

Orange: Social and Fun. An energizing, lively, and invigorating warm color that evokes enthusiasm, self-confidence, and creativity.

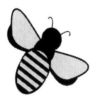

Yellow: Cheerful and Playful. It rejuvenates and stimulates your mind, body, and soul while sparking imagination and innovation. It epitomizes warmth and an optimistic outlook to the future.

Dark Green: Calm and Reassuring; **Bright Green:** Youthful and Naïve. Green is a very popular color due in part to its calming and restful effect. Varying shades of green evoke a stable and secure environment by creating a sense of balance and harmony. It is a cool, nurturing color that promotes healing and regrowth.

Blue: Friendly, Safe, and Secure. Blue represents communication, reliability, peace, tranquility and truth. An intellectual color that evokes a protective mood, it symbolizes loyalty and control.

Indigo/Violet/Purple: Creative and Unconventional. The color promotes spirituality and intuition. It defines elegance and refined luxury. Representing a sense of power and royalty, it suggests wealth and sophistication.

Light Pink: Soft and Nurturing; **Bright Pink:** Confident, assured, and provides a temporary calming effect. Think of this as bubble gum pink. This is a short-term effect, as the body always strives for "balance." When the hue becomes too bold, it is more attractive to men than to women. Consider your audience when you wear pink.

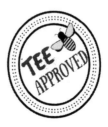

Maintain an Interesting Appearance - It Matters

Nothing explains who we are and what we're all about better than style and fashion. Style matters. Fashion is important. You know it when you see it; someone enters a room, and you say to yourself, "He has style," or "That is someone I want to meet." It's an energy that is undeniable, a confidence you can feel. Not everyone has "it." Not everyone does "it" authentically.

As an example: When buying an outfit off a mannequin, you don't need to wonder if the pieces go together because someone in the store already put it together. It's easy. You might find the outfit appealing, but that doesn't mean it represents the true you. If you are not the same shape or size as the mannequin, it won't fit you the same.

I find many people dress blandly. Men do this often—for instance, a polo and khakis with boat shoes—bland, typical, doesn't say much about them. The "safe" dressing for women that I see most often is the all-black default. For example, in the last month I've been the guest in several new closets with all black shoes: black sandals, athletic shoes, pumps, and wedges—not very interesting, just safe.

Most people play it safe when shopping. They try to work themselves out of that safe, bland box, but without individual guidance and advice that is specific to their body and lifestyle, they fall short and flat. Often, I can show them how to create a more interesting image without shopping. It all begins with how items are paired or layered.

Just yesterday, I worked with a plus-size 60-year-old businesswoman. Using items she already owned, some clothes pins, a belt I had in my tote bag, and a necklace she had shoved away in a drawer and had never worn, I made her look interesting. I focused on teaching her the right proportion for her 5-foot-3 frame. I created a waist that wasn't previously visible. I pushed up her sleeves and visually sliced her in half with a pop of color, a print worn in just the right place. She looked ageless, modern, approachable, and professional. How perfect! Those were the very style words she had written down before I arrived.

I showed the client why the neckline she had invested heavily into wasn't flattering in any way. I demonstrated how fabulous her legs were when wearing skirts hemmed to her "sweet spot." Oh my! we had some "ah-ha" moments. Now she can't wait to shop with me so we can flesh out her new fresh look.

Helpful tips to show men how to appear more interesting:
- Try on a suit vest and wear with jeans.
- Add a pocket square that contrasts your tie.
- Roll you jean hem up a little and don't wear socks.
- Buy some denim lace-up shoes.
- Pop some color other than living in black or navy.

Helpful tips to show women how to appear more interesting:
- If you always wear pants, get into a skirt or dress or try a jumpsuit.
- Ditch black shoes for the entire summer and wear metallic, nude or color instead.
- Don't always wear the same tiny earrings and small-scale necklace. Go up a size or try a statement necklace or earrings (but not at the same time)
- Try something new; a scarf, hat, belt, or colored purse.

Harness Your Superpowers!

We all have superpowers, yet we don't always maximize them. Think in terms of your personal image. What sets you apart from the people around you? Do you have great posture, a quick smile, and mindful body language? Perhaps you have impeccable manners or are easily able to build rapport with others.

Most people, especially women, have difficulty being objective about themselves. As I spend time with individuals in their closets or dressing rooms, I find that many are unaware of their superpower, so when I point out something about them, they are shocked as if they never considered it a plus.

So what is your special superpower? It could be something physical, such as shapely legs, big eyes, a strong jaw line, or some other feature. If so, play it up, not in an overtly sexy way but with a nice balance to your overall look.

I know several people who have excellent recall of names and details people have shared with them in casual conversations. I'm not good at that at all, and I admire them for that superpower, which motivates me to practice that trait. Have you ever met someone with whom, for some compelling reason, you want to reveal details that you just wouldn't normally offer? It's probably because they have a superpower of a trusting energy.

Think of this: I know a photographer who can easily and quickly coax the best and truest of her muse out of a child or adult. Superpower!

I met an insurance agent who radiated honesty and knowledge. Rather than being a sales person who is selling a product, she is able to guide an individual to make the best choices to protect their dreams. Superpower!

My superpower is seeing clients' wardrobes and putting them at ease in the most intimate setting—their closet—while expressing no judgment yet teaching them how to elevate their style.

How can you harness your superpower while appreciating the superpowers of others? Do you know people who might have the superpowers of compassion, creativity, intuition, bravery or empathy? Some of us are blessed with more of these traits than others. Use them to lift others and make others feel, loved, heard, appreciated, and valued.

Love Yourself at Every Size and Dress your Now Body

Don't wait to lose weight before updating your wardrobe. I often hear people tell me that when they lose weight they will invest in their wardrobe. I'm suggesting that you dress your best each and every day to keep your energy and goals more focused. Use these tips to trick the eye and play-up your best assets.

Look your best now, and even 10 or 20 pounds from now, by focusing the attention where you want it. Use the clothes as the tools they are. Harness the power of your wardrobe.

Are you still struggling to make sense of your wardrobe? Are your closet and drawers full, yet you're paralyzed when trying to decide what to give away and what to keep or tailor?

Stop the madness and create a step by step plan. Rarely should anyone pitch everything and begin from scratch. Always begin with a "Closet Detox," never a trip to the stores. Take action now for a streamlined and effortless daily routine that puts your best self into the world every day.

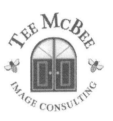

MASTERING YOUR EVOLVING STYLE

Second Edition

30-DAY WARDROBE PLANNING JOURNAL

Let's Begin!

DATE: _____ **DAY:** M T W TH F SAT SUN

YOUR MOOD: _____

WHO IS YOUR AUDIENCE?   (CIRCLE)

SHOPPING/ERRANDS   DOCTORS (SELF/KIDS)   TRAVEL

KIDS EVENTS   FAMILY FUNCTION   SINGLES EVENT

PROF. MEETINGS   CASUAL WORK DAY   HOME OFFICE DAY

FACE/FACE MEETING   ON-SITE CLIENT MEETING

NETWORKING   VIDEO CONFERENCE   PRESENTATION

DATE NIGHT   PARTY: CASUAL OR DRESSY   GIRLS NIGHT

HOLIDAY /SPECIAL EVENT   _____

_____   _____   _____

WHAT GOAL / MESSAGE ARE YOU COMMUNICATING ?
(BUSINESS AND OR PERSONAL)

BUILDING RAPPORT / TRUST   CONFIDENT / SELF–ASSURED

LEADER   INDEPENDENT / SELF-SUFFICIENT

FASCINATING / INTRIGING   EDUCATE / TEACH

CHARMING / ENGAGING   ALLURING / ROMANTIC

WEATHER:

RAIN   SNOW   SUNNY   HOT   HUMID

SPRING COLD/WARM   SUMMER COOL/HOT   FALL COLD/WARM

WINTER COLD/WARM   UMBRELLA   RAINCOAT

BACK UP SHOES   BOOTS / TRACK SHOES   _____

WHICH STYLE WORDS ARE YOU COMMUNICATING?

CONFIDENT   PROFESSIONAL   POWERFUL   SEXY   FUN

SAVVY   FRESH   MODERN   APPROACHABLE   AGELESS

PUT-TOGETHER   TRENDY   IN-CONTROL   WHIMSICAL

_____   _____   _____

MAIN WARDROBE EVENT: _____

TODAY'S OUTFIT   (REFER TO LOOK BOOK)

MAINTENANCE / UPKEEP

SNIFF TEST: DRY CLEANERS? CHECK SHOES?

DAMAGE/REPAIRS NEEDED   (PUT IN SPECIAL PLACE)

END OF DAY OUTFIT REVIEW

HOW DID YOU FEEL? DID YOU GET COMPLIMENTS?
DID YOU REACH YOUR GOAL TODAY?

DATE: _____ **DAY:** M T W TH F SAT SUN

YOUR MOOD: _____

WHO IS YOUR AUDIENCE? (CIRCLE)

SHOPPING/ERRANDS   DOCTORS (SELF/KIDS)   TRAVEL

KIDS EVENTS   FAMILY FUNCTION   SINGLES EVENT

PROF. MEETINGS   CASUAL WORK DAY   HOME OFFICE DAY

FACE/FACE MEETING   ON-SITE CLIENT MEETING

NETWORKING   VIDEO CONFERENCE   PRESENTATION

DATE NIGHT   PARTY: CASUAL OR DRESSY   GIRLS NIGHT

HOLIDAY /SPECIAL EVENT   _____

_____   _____   _____

WHAT GOAL / MESSAGE ARE YOU COMMUNICATING ?
(BUSINESS AND OR PERSONAL)

BUILDING RAPPORT / TRUST   CONFIDENT / SELF-ASSURED

LEADER   INDEPENDENT / SELF-SUFFICIENT

FASCINATING / INTRIGING   EDUCATE / TEACH

CHARMING / ENGAGING   ALLURING / ROMANTIC

WEATHER:

RAIN   SNOW   SUNNY   HOT   HUMID

SPRING COLD/WARM   SUMMER COOL/HOT   FALL COLD/WARM

WINTER COLD/WARM   UMBRELLA   RAINCOAT

BACK UP SHOES   BOOTS / TRACK SHOES   _____

WHICH STYLE WORDS ARE YOU COMMUNICATING?

CONFIDENT   PROFESSIONAL POWERFUL   SEXY   FUN

SAVVY   FRESH   MODERN   APPROACHABLE   AGELESS

PUT-TOGETHER   TRENDY   IN-CONTROL   WHIMSICAL

_____   _____   _____

MAIN WARDROBE EVENT: _____

TODAY'S OUTFIT   (REFER TO LOOK BOOK)

-------------------------   -------------------------
-------------------------   -------------------------
-------------------------   -------------------------
-------------------------   -------------------------
-------------------------   -------------------------
-------------------------   -------------------------
-------------------------   -------------------------

MAINTENANCE / UPKEEP

SNIFF TEST: DRY CLEANERS? CHECK SHOES?

DAMAGE/REPAIRS NEEDED   (PUT IN SPECIAL PLACE)

-------------------------   -------------------------
-------------------------   -------------------------
-------------------------   -------------------------
-------------------------   -------------------------
-------------------------   -------------------------

END OF DAY OUTFIT REVIEW

HOW DID YOU FEEL? DID YOU GET COMPLIMENTS?
DID YOU REACH YOUR GOAL TODAY?

_____
_____
_____
_____
_____
_____

DATE: _____ DAY: M T W TH F SAT SUN

YOUR MOOD: _____

WHO IS YOUR AUDIENCE?   (CIRCLE)

SHOPPING/ERRANDS   DOCTORS (SELF/KIDS)   TRAVEL

KIDS EVENTS   FAMILY FUNCTION   SINGLES EVENT

PROF. MEETINGS   CASUAL WORK DAY   HOME OFFICE DAY

FACE/FACE MEETING   ON-SITE CLIENT MEETING

NETWORKING   VIDEO CONFERENCE   PRESENTATION

DATE NIGHT   PARTY: CASUAL OR DRESSY   GIRLS NIGHT

HOLIDAY /SPECIAL EVENT   _____

_____   _____   _____

WHAT GOAL / MESSAGE ARE YOU COMMUNICATING ?
(BUSINESS AND OR PERSONAL)

BUILDING RAPPORT / TRUST   CONFIDENT / SELF-ASSURED

LEADER   INDEPENDENT / SELF-SUFFICIENT

FASCINATING / INTRIGING   EDUCATE / TEACH

CHARMING / ENGAGING   ALLURING / ROMANTIC

WEATHER:

RAIN   SNOW   SUNNY   HOT   HUMID

SPRING COLD/WARM   SUMMER COOL/HOT   FALL COLD/WARM

WINTER COLD/WARM   UMBRELLA   RAINCOAT

BACK UP SHOES   BOOTS / TRACK SHOES   _____

WHICH STYLE WORDS ARE YOU COMMUNICATING?

CONFIDENT   PROFESSIONAL POWERFUL   SEXY   FUN

SAVVY   FRESH   MODERN   APPROACHABLE   AGELESS

PUT-TOGETHER   TRENDY   IN-CONTROL   WHIMSICAL

_____   _____   _____

MAIN WARDROBE EVENT: _____

TODAY'S OUTFIT   (REFER TO LOOK BOOK)

_____   _____

_____   _____

_____   _____

_____   _____

_____   _____

_____   _____

_____   _____

MAINTENANCE / UPKEEP

SNIFF TEST: DRY CLEANERS? CHECK SHOES?

DAMAGE/REPAIRS NEEDED   (PUT IN SPECIAL PLACE)

_____   _____

_____   _____

_____   _____

_____   _____

_____   _____

END OF DAY OUTFIT REVIEW

HOW DID YOU FEEL? DID YOU GET COMPLIMENTS?
DID YOU REACH YOUR GOAL TODAY?

_____

_____

_____

_____

_____

_____

DATE: _____ **DAY:** M T W TH F SAT SUN

YOUR MOOD: _____

WHO IS YOUR AUDIENCE? (CIRCLE)

SHOPPING/ERRANDS   DOCTORS (SELF/KIDS)   TRAVEL

KIDS EVENTS   FAMILY FUNCTION   SINGLES EVENT

PROF. MEETINGS   CASUAL WORK DAY   HOME OFFICE DAY

FACE/FACE MEETING   ON-SITE CLIENT MEETING

NETWORKING   VIDEO CONFERENCE   PRESENTATION

DATE NIGHT   PARTY: CASUAL OR DRESSY   GIRLS NIGHT

HOLIDAY /SPECIAL EVENT   _____

_____   _____   _____

WHAT GOAL / MESSAGE ARE YOU COMMUNICATING ?
(BUSINESS AND OR PERSONAL)

BUILDING RAPPORT / TRUST   CONFIDENT / SELF-ASSURED

LEADER   INDEPENDENT / SELF-SUFFICIENT

FASCINATING / INTRIGING   EDUCATE / TEACH

CHARMING / ENGAGING   ALLURING / ROMANTIC

WEATHER:

RAIN   SNOW   SUNNY   HOT   HUMID

SPRING COLD/WARM   SUMMER COOL/HOT   FALL COLD/WARM

WINTER COLD/WARM   UMBRELLA   RAINCOAT

BACK UP SHOES   BOOTS / TRACK SHOES   _____

WHICH STYLE WORDS ARE YOU COMMUNICATING?

CONFIDENT   PROFESSIONAL POWERFUL   SEXY   FUN

SAVVY   FRESH   MODERN   APPROACHABLE   AGELESS

PUT-TOGETHER   TRENDY   IN-CONTROL   WHIMSICAL

_____   _____   _____

MAIN WARDROBE EVENT: _____

TODAY'S OUTFIT (REFER TO LOOK BOOK)

---------------------------------   ---------------------------------
---------------------------------   ---------------------------------
---------------------------------   ---------------------------------
---------------------------------   ---------------------------------
---------------------------------   ---------------------------------
---------------------------------   ---------------------------------

MAINTENANCE / UPKEEP

SNIFF TEST: DRY CLEANERS? CHECK SHOES?

DAMAGE/REPAIRS NEEDED (PUT IN SPECIAL PLACE)

---------------------------------   ---------------------------------
---------------------------------   ---------------------------------
---------------------------------   ---------------------------------
---------------------------------   ---------------------------------

END OF DAY OUTFIT REVIEW

HOW DID YOU FEEL? DID YOU GET COMPLIMENTS?
DID YOU REACH YOUR GOAL TODAY?

_____
_____
_____
_____
_____
_____

If you know you're going after work to see your gynecologist, don't wear panty hose and a dress to work that day. Wear slacks something easy to slip on and slip off. **Dress for your audience** so, in this case, **your gynecologists**!

At the end of the day look closely at your shoes, are they scuffed? Need to be wiped down? Or cleaned?

Make sure you **mark it on your log** that it needs maintenance.

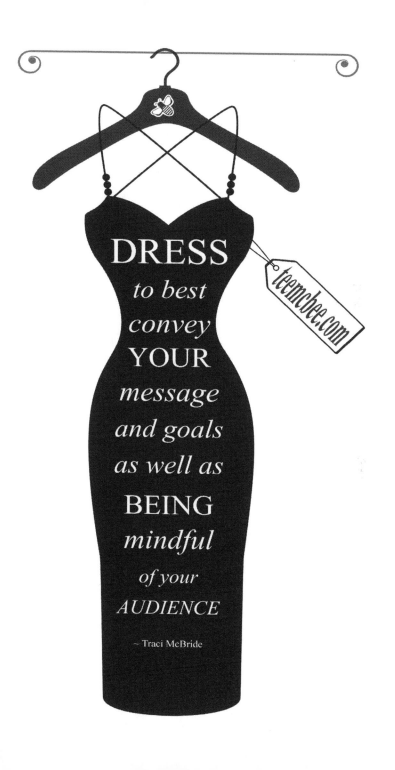

DRESS *to best convey* YOUR *message and goals as well as* BEING *mindful of your* AUDIENCE

~ Traci McBride

DATE: _____ **DAY:** M T W TH F SAT SUN

YOUR MOOD: _____

WHO IS YOUR AUDIENCE?   (CIRCLE)

SHOPPING/ERRANDS   DOCTORS (SELF/KIDS)   TRAVEL

KIDS EVENTS   FAMILY FUNCTION   SINGLES EVENT

PROF. MEETINGS   CASUAL WORK DAY   HOME OFFICE DAY

FACE/FACE MEETING   ON-SITE CLIENT MEETING

NETWORKING   VIDEO CONFERENCE   PRESENTATION

DATE NIGHT   PARTY: CASUAL OR DRESSY   GIRLS NIGHT

HOLIDAY /SPECIAL EVENT   _____

_____   _____   _____

WHAT GOAL / MESSAGE ARE YOU COMMUNICATING ?
(BUSINESS AND OR PERSONAL)

BUILDING RAPPORT / TRUST   CONFIDENT / SELF-ASSURED

LEADER   INDEPENDENT / SELF-SUFFICIENT

FASCINATING / INTRIGING   EDUCATE / TEACH

CHARMING / ENGAGING   ALLURING / ROMANTIC

WEATHER:

RAIN   SNOW   SUNNY   HOT   HUMID

SPRING COLD/WARM   SUMMER COOL/HOT   FALL COLD/WARM

WINTER COLD/WARM   UMBRELLA   RAINCOAT

BACK UP SHOES   BOOTS / TRACK SHOES   _____

WHICH STYLE WORDS ARE YOU COMMUNICATING?

CONFIDENT   PROFESSIONAL POWERFUL   SEXY   FUN

SAVVY   FRESH   MODERN   APPROACHABLE   AGELESS

PUT-TOGETHER   TRENDY   IN-CONTROL   WHIMSICAL

_____   _____   _____

MAIN WARDROBE EVENT: _____

TODAY'S OUTFIT   (REFER TO LOOK BOOK)

_____   _____
_____   _____
_____   _____
_____   _____
_____   _____
_____   _____
_____   _____

MAINTENANCE / UPKEEP

SNIFF TEST: DRY CLEANERS? CHECK SHOES?

DAMAGE/REPAIRS NEEDED   (PUT IN SPECIAL PLACE)

_____   _____
_____   _____
_____   _____
_____   _____

END OF DAY OUTFIT REVIEW

HOW DID YOU FEEL? DID YOU GET COMPLIMENTS?
DID YOU REACH YOUR GOAL TODAY?

_____
_____
_____
_____
_____
_____
_____

DATE: _____ **DAY:** M T W TH F SAT SUN

YOUR MOOD: _____

WHO IS YOUR AUDIENCE?   (CIRCLE)

SHOPPING/ERRANDS   DOCTORS (SELF/KIDS)   TRAVEL

KIDS EVENTS   FAMILY FUNCTION   SINGLES EVENT

PROF. MEETINGS   CASUAL WORK DAY   HOME OFFICE DAY

FACE/FACE MEETING   ON-SITE CLIENT MEETING

NETWORKING   VIDEO CONFERENCE   PRESENTATION

DATE NIGHT   PARTY: CASUAL OR DRESSY   GIRLS NIGHT

HOLIDAY /SPECIAL EVENT   _____

_____   _____   _____

WHAT GOAL / MESSAGE ARE YOU COMMUNICATING ?
(BUSINESS AND OR PERSONAL)

BUILDING RAPPORT / TRUST   CONFIDENT / SELF-ASSURED

LEADER   INDEPENDENT / SELF-SUFFICIENT

FASCINATING / INTRIGING   EDUCATE / TEACH

CHARMING / ENGAGING   ALLURING / ROMANTIC

WEATHER:

RAIN   SNOW   SUNNY   HOT   HUMID

SPRING COLD/WARM   SUMMER COOL/HOT   FALL COLD/WARM

WINTER COLD/WARM   UMBRELLA   RAINCOAT

BACK UP SHOES   BOOTS / TRACK SHOES   _____

WHICH STYLE WORDS ARE YOU COMMUNICATING?

CONFIDENT   PROFESSIONAL POWERFUL   SEXY   FUN

SAVVY   FRESH   MODERN   APPROACHABLE   AGELESS

PUT-TOGETHER   TRENDY   IN-CONTROL   WHIMSICAL

_____   _____   _____

MAIN WARDROBE EVENT: _____

TODAY'S OUTFIT (REFER TO LOOK BOOK)

---------------------------   ---------------------------
---------------------------   ---------------------------
---------------------------   ---------------------------
---------------------------   ---------------------------
---------------------------   ---------------------------
---------------------------   ---------------------------
---------------------------   ---------------------------

MAINTENANCE / UPKEEP
SNIFF TEST: DRY CLEANERS? CHECK SHOES?

DAMAGE/REPAIRS NEEDED   (PUT IN SPECIAL PLACE)

---------------------------   ---------------------------
---------------------------   ---------------------------
---------------------------   ---------------------------
---------------------------   ---------------------------
---------------------------   ---------------------------

END OF DAY OUTFIT REVIEW
HOW DID YOU FEEL? DID YOU GET COMPLIMENTS?
DID YOU REACH YOUR GOAL TODAY?

_____

_____

_____

_____

_____

_____

DATE: _____ DAY: M T W TH F SAT SUN

YOUR MOOD: _____

WHO IS YOUR AUDIENCE? (CIRCLE)

SHOPPING/ERRANDS   DOCTORS (SELF/KIDS)   TRAVEL

KIDS EVENTS   FAMILY FUNCTION   SINGLES EVENT

PROF. MEETINGS   CASUAL WORK DAY   HOME OFFICE DAY

FACE/FACE MEETING   ON-SITE CLIENT MEETING

NETWORKING   VIDEO CONFERENCE   PRESENTATION

DATE NIGHT   PARTY: CASUAL OR DRESSY   GIRLS NIGHT

HOLIDAY /SPECIAL EVENT   _____

_____   _____   _____

WHAT GOAL / MESSAGE ARE YOU COMMUNICATING ?
(BUSINESS AND OR PERSONAL)

BUILDING RAPPORT / TRUST   CONFIDENT / SELF-ASSURED

LEADER   INDEPENDENT / SELF-SUFFICIENT

FASCINATING / INTRIGING   EDUCATE / TEACH

CHARMING / ENGAGING   ALLURING / ROMANTIC

WEATHER:

RAIN   SNOW   SUNNY   HOT   HUMID

SPRING COLD/WARM   SUMMER COOL/HOT   FALL COLD/WARM

WINTER COLD/WARM   UMBRELLA   RAINCOAT

BACK UP SHOES   BOOTS / TRACK SHOES   _____

WHICH STYLE WORDS ARE YOU COMMUNICATING?

CONFIDENT   PROFESSIONAL POWERFUL   SEXY   FUN

SAVVY   FRESH   MODERN   APPROACHABLE   AGELESS

PUT-TOGETHER   TRENDY   IN-CONTROL   WHIMSICAL

_____   _____   _____

MAIN WARDROBE EVENT: _____

TODAY'S OUTFIT   (REFER TO LOOK BOOK)

_____   _____

_____   _____

_____   _____

_____   _____

_____   _____

_____   _____

_____   _____

MAINTENANCE / UPKEEP

SNIFF TEST: DRY CLEANERS? CHECK SHOES?

DAMAGE/REPAIRS NEEDED   (PUT IN SPECIAL PLACE)

_____   _____

_____   _____

_____   _____

_____   _____

END OF DAY OUTFIT REVIEW

HOW DID YOU FEEL? DID YOU GET COMPLIMENTS?
DID YOU REACH YOUR GOAL TODAY?

_____

_____

_____

_____

_____

_____

DATE: _____ **DAY:** M T W TH F SAT SUN

YOUR MOOD: _____

WHO IS YOUR AUDIENCE?   (CIRCLE)

SHOPPING/ERRANDS   DOCTORS (SELF/KIDS)   TRAVEL

KIDS EVENTS   FAMILY FUNCTION   SINGLES EVENT

PROF. MEETINGS   CASUAL WORK DAY   HOME OFFICE DAY

FACE/FACE MEETING   ON-SITE CLIENT MEETING

NETWORKING   VIDEO CONFERENCE   PRESENTATION

DATE NIGHT   PARTY: CASUAL OR DRESSY   GIRLS NIGHT

HOLIDAY /SPECIAL EVENT   _____

_____   _____   _____

WHAT GOAL / MESSAGE ARE YOU COMMUNICATING ?
(BUSINESS AND OR PERSONAL)

BUILDING RAPPORT / TRUST   CONFIDENT / SELF-ASSURED

LEADER   INDEPENDENT / SELF-SUFFICIENT

FASCINATING / INTRIGING   EDUCATE / TEACH

CHARMING / ENGAGING   ALLURING / ROMANTIC

WEATHER:

RAIN   SNOW   SUNNY   HOT   HUMID

SPRING COLD/WARM   SUMMER COOL/HOT   FALL COLD/WARM

WINTER COLD/WARM   UMBRELLA   RAINCOAT

BACK UP SHOES   BOOTS / TRACK SHOES   _____

WHICH STYLE WORDS ARE YOU COMMUNICATING?

CONFIDENT   PROFESSIONAL   POWERFUL   SEXY   FUN

SAVVY   FRESH   MODERN   APPROACHABLE   AGELESS

PUT-TOGETHER   TRENDY   IN-CONTROL   WHIMSICAL

_____   _____   _____

MAIN WARDROBE EVENT: _____

TODAY'S OUTFIT   (REFER TO LOOK BOOK)

_____   _____
_____   _____
_____   _____
_____   _____
_____   _____
_____   _____

MAINTENANCE / UPKEEP

SNIFF TEST: DRY CLEANERS? CHECK SHOES?

DAMAGE/REPAIRS NEEDED   (PUT IN SPECIAL PLACE)

_____   _____
_____   _____
_____   _____
_____   _____

END OF DAY OUTFIT REVIEW

HOW DID YOU FEEL? DID YOU GET COMPLIMENTS?
DID YOU REACH YOUR GOAL TODAY?

_____
_____
_____
_____
_____
_____

What do YOU want people to assume or think of you at a glance?

Dress with your chosen message
EVERY DAY.

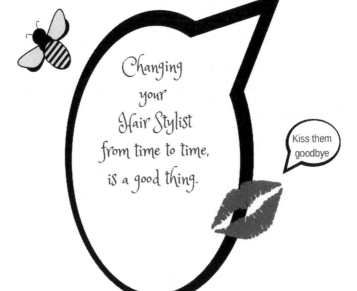

Changing
your
Hair Stylist
from time to time,
is a good thing.

Kiss them
goodbye

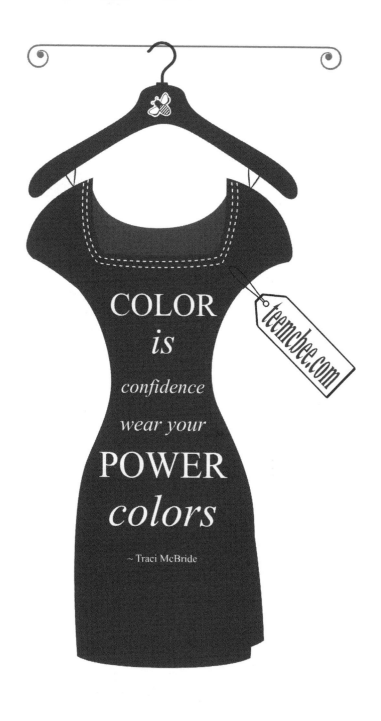

COLOR *is* confidence wear your POWER *colors*

~ Traci McBride

DATE: _____ **DAY:** M T W TH F SAT SUN

YOUR MOOD: _____

WHO IS YOUR AUDIENCE?   (CIRCLE)

SHOPPING/ERRANDS   DOCTORS (SELF/KIDS)   TRAVEL

KIDS EVENTS   FAMILY FUNCTION   SINGLES EVENT

PROF. MEETINGS   CASUAL WORK DAY   HOME OFFICE DAY

FACE/FACE MEETING   ON-SITE CLIENT MEETING

NETWORKING   VIDEO CONFERENCE   PRESENTATION

DATE NIGHT   PARTY: CASUAL OR DRESSY   GIRLS NIGHT

HOLIDAY /SPECIAL EVENT   _____

_____   _____   _____

WHAT GOAL / MESSAGE ARE YOU COMMUNICATING ?
(BUSINESS AND OR PERSONAL)

BUILDING RAPPORT / TRUST   CONFIDENT / SELF-ASSURED

LEADER   INDEPENDENT / SELF-SUFFICIENT

FASCINATING / INTRIGING   EDUCATE / TEACH

CHARMING / ENGAGING   ALLURING / ROMANTIC

WEATHER:

RAIN   SNOW   SUNNY   HOT   HUMID

SPRING COLD/WARM   SUMMER COOL/HOT   FALL COLD/WARM

WINTER COLD/WARM   UMBRELLA   RAINCOAT

BACK UP SHOES   BOOTS / TRACK SHOES   _____

WHICH STYLE WORDS ARE YOU COMMUNICATING?

CONFIDENT   PROFESSIONAL   POWERFUL   SEXY   FUN

SAVVY   FRESH   MODERN   APPROACHABLE   AGELESS

PUT-TOGETHER   TRENDY   IN-CONTROL   WHIMSICAL

_____   _____   _____

MAIN WARDROBE EVENT: _____

TODAY'S OUTFIT   (REFER TO LOOK BOOK)

_____   _____
_____   _____
_____   _____
_____   _____
_____   _____
_____   _____
_____   _____

MAINTENANCE / UPKEEP

SNIFF TEST: DRY CLEANERS? CHECK SHOES?

DAMAGE/REPAIRS NEEDED   (PUT IN SPECIAL PLACE)

_____   _____
_____   _____
_____   _____
_____   _____

END OF DAY OUTFIT REVIEW

HOW DID YOU FEEL? DID YOU GET COMPLIMENTS?
DID YOU REACH YOUR GOAL TODAY?

_____
_____
_____
_____
_____
_____

DATE: _____ DAY: M T W TH F SAT SUN

YOUR MOOD: _____

WHO IS YOUR AUDIENCE? (CIRCLE)

SHOPPING/ERRANDS   DOCTORS (SELF/KIDS)   TRAVEL

KIDS EVENTS   FAMILY FUNCTION   SINGLES EVENT

PROF. MEETINGS   CASUAL WORK DAY   HOME OFFICE DAY

FACE/FACE MEETING   ON-SITE CLIENT MEETING

NETWORKING   VIDEO CONFERENCE   PRESENTATION

DATE NIGHT   PARTY: CASUAL OR DRESSY   GIRLS NIGHT

HOLIDAY /SPECIAL EVENT   _____

_____   _____   _____

WHAT GOAL / MESSAGE ARE YOU COMMUNICATING ?
(BUSINESS AND OR PERSONAL)

BUILDING RAPPORT / TRUST   CONFIDENT / SELF-ASSURED

LEADER   INDEPENDENT / SELF-SUFFICIENT

FASCINATING / INTRIGING   EDUCATE / TEACH

CHARMING / ENGAGING   ALLURING / ROMANTIC

WEATHER:

RAIN   SNOW   SUNNY   HOT   HUMID

SPRING COLD/WARM   SUMMER COOL/HOT   FALL COLD/WARM

WINTER COLD/WARM   UMBRELLA   RAINCOAT

BACK UP SHOES   BOOTS / TRACK SHOES   _____

WHICH STYLE WORDS ARE YOU COMMUNICATING?

CONFIDENT   PROFESSIONAL POWERFUL   SEXY   FUN

SAVVY   FRESH   MODERN   APPROACHABLE   AGELESS

PUT-TOGETHER   TRENDY   IN-CONTROL   WHIMSICAL

_____   _____   _____

MAIN WARDROBE EVENT: _____

TODAY'S OUTFIT   (REFER TO LOOK BOOK)

_____   _____
_____   _____
_____   _____
_____   _____
_____   _____
_____   _____
_____   _____

MAINTENANCE / UPKEEP

SNIFF TEST: DRY CLEANERS? CHECK SHOES?

DAMAGE/REPAIRS NEEDED   (PUT IN SPECIAL PLACE)

_____   _____
_____   _____
_____   _____
_____   _____
_____   _____

END OF DAY OUTFIT REVIEW

HOW DID YOU FEEL? DID YOU GET COMPLIMENTS?
DID YOU REACH YOUR GOAL TODAY?

_____
_____
_____
_____
_____
_____
_____

DATE: _____ DAY: M T W TH F SAT SUN

YOUR MOOD: _____

WHO IS YOUR AUDIENCE?   (CIRCLE)

SHOPPING/ERRANDS   DOCTORS (SELF/KIDS)   TRAVEL

KIDS EVENTS   FAMILY FUNCTION   SINGLES EVENT

PROF. MEETINGS   CASUAL WORK DAY   HOME OFFICE DAY

FACE/FACE MEETING   ON-SITE CLIENT MEETING

NETWORKING   VIDEO CONFERENCE   PRESENTATION

DATE NIGHT   PARTY: CASUAL OR DRESSY   GIRLS NIGHT

HOLIDAY /SPECIAL EVENT   _____

_____   _____   _____

WHAT GOAL / MESSAGE ARE YOU COMMUNICATING ?
(BUSINESS AND OR PERSONAL)

BUILDING RAPPORT / TRUST   CONFIDENT / SELF-ASSURED

LEADER   INDEPENDENT / SELF-SUFFICIENT

FASCINATING / INTRIGING   EDUCATE / TEACH

CHARMING / ENGAGING   ALLURING / ROMANTIC

WEATHER:

RAIN   SNOW   SUNNY   HOT   HUMID

SPRING COLD/WARM   SUMMER COOL/HOT   FALL COLD/WARM

WINTER COLD/WARM   UMBRELLA   RAINCOAT

BACK UP SHOES   BOOTS / TRACK SHOES   _____

WHICH STYLE WORDS ARE YOU COMMUNICATING?

CONFIDENT   PROFESSIONAL POWERFUL   SEXY   FUN

SAVVY   FRESH   MODERN   APPROACHABLE   AGELESS

PUT-TOGETHER   TRENDY   IN-CONTROL   WHIMSICAL

_____   _____   _____

MAIN WARDROBE EVENT: _____

TODAY'S OUTFIT   (REFER TO LOOK BOOK)

_____   _____
_____   _____
_____   _____
_____   _____
_____   _____
_____   _____
_____   _____
_____   _____

MAINTENANCE / UPKEEP

SNIFF TEST: DRY CLEANERS? CHECK SHOES?

DAMAGE/REPAIRS NEEDED   (PUT IN SPECIAL PLACE)

_____   _____
_____   _____
_____   _____
_____   _____
_____   _____

END OF DAY OUTFIT REVIEW

HOW DID YOU FEEL? DID YOU GET COMPLIMENTS?
DID YOU REACH YOUR GOAL TODAY?

_____
_____
_____
_____
_____
_____
_____

DATE: _____ DAY: M T W TH F SAT SUN

YOUR MOOD: _____

WHO IS YOUR AUDIENCE? (CIRCLE)

SHOPPING/ERRANDS   DOCTORS (SELF/KIDS)   TRAVEL

KIDS EVENTS   FAMILY FUNCTION   SINGLES EVENT

PROF. MEETINGS   CASUAL WORK DAY   HOME OFFICE DAY

FACE/FACE MEETING   ON-SITE CLIENT MEETING

NETWORKING   VIDEO CONFERENCE   PRESENTATION

DATE NIGHT   PARTY: CASUAL OR DRESSY   GIRLS NIGHT

HOLIDAY /SPECIAL EVENT   _____

_____   _____   _____

WHAT GOAL / MESSAGE ARE YOU COMMUNICATING ?
(BUSINESS AND OR PERSONAL)

BUILDING RAPPORT / TRUST   CONFIDENT / SELF-ASSURED

LEADER   INDEPENDENT / SELF-SUFFICIENT

FASCINATING / INTRIGING   EDUCATE / TEACH

CHARMING / ENGAGING   ALLURING / ROMANTIC

WEATHER:

RAIN   SNOW   SUNNY   HOT   HUMID

SPRING COLD/WARM   SUMMER COOL/HOT   FALL COLD/WARM

WINTER COLD/WARM   UMBRELLA   RAINCOAT

BACK UP SHOES   BOOTS / TRACK SHOES   _____

WHICH STYLE WORDS ARE YOU COMMUNICATING?

CONFIDENT   PROFESSIONAL POWERFUL   SEXY   FUN

SAVVY   FRESH   MODERN   APPROACHABLE   AGELESS

PUT-TOGETHER   TRENDY   IN-CONTROL   WHIMSICAL

_____   _____   _____

MAIN WARDROBE EVENT: _____

TODAY'S OUTFIT   (REFER TO LOOK BOOK)

----------------------------   ----------------------------
----------------------------   ----------------------------
----------------------------   ----------------------------
----------------------------   ----------------------------
----------------------------   ----------------------------
----------------------------   ----------------------------
----------------------------   ----------------------------

MAINTENANCE / UPKEEP

SNIFF TEST: DRY CLEANERS? CHECK SHOES?

DAMAGE/REPAIRS NEEDED   (PUT IN SPECIAL PLACE)

----------------------------   ----------------------------
----------------------------   ----------------------------
----------------------------   ----------------------------
----------------------------   ----------------------------
----------------------------   ----------------------------

END OF DAY OUTFIT REVIEW

HOW DID YOU FEEL? DID YOU GET COMPLIMENTS?
DID YOU REACH YOUR GOAL TODAY?

_____
_____
_____
_____
_____
_____

DATE: _____ **DAY:** M T W TH F SAT SUN

YOUR MOOD: _____

WHO IS YOUR AUDIENCE?   (CIRCLE)

SHOPPING/ERRANDS   DOCTORS (SELF/KIDS)   TRAVEL

KIDS EVENTS   FAMILY FUNCTION   SINGLES EVENT

PROF. MEETINGS   CASUAL WORK DAY   HOME OFFICE DAY

FACE/FACE MEETING   ON-SITE CLIENT MEETING

NETWORKING   VIDEO CONFERENCE   PRESENTATION

DATE NIGHT   PARTY: CASUAL OR DRESSY   GIRLS NIGHT

HOLIDAY /SPECIAL EVENT   _____

_____   _____   _____

WHAT GOAL / MESSAGE ARE YOU COMMUNICATING ?
(BUSINESS AND OR PERSONAL)

BUILDING RAPPORT / TRUST   CONFIDENT / SELF-ASSURED

LEADER   INDEPENDENT / SELF-SUFFICIENT

FASCINATING / INTRIGING   EDUCATE / TEACH

CHARMING / ENGAGING   ALLURING / ROMANTIC

WEATHER:

RAIN   SNOW   SUNNY   HOT   HUMID

SPRING COLD/WARM   SUMMER COOL/HOT   FALL COLD/WARM

WINTER COLD/WARM   UMBRELLA   RAINCOAT

BACK UP SHOES   BOOTS / TRACK SHOES   _____

WHICH STYLE WORDS ARE YOU COMMUNICATING?

CONFIDENT   PROFESSIONAL POWERFUL   SEXY   FUN

SAVVY   FRESH   MODERN   APPROACHABLE   AGELESS

PUT-TOGETHER   TRENDY   IN-CONTROL   WHIMSICAL

_____   _____   _____

MAIN WARDROBE EVENT: _____

TODAY'S OUTFIT   (REFER TO LOOK BOOK)

_____   _____
_____   _____
_____   _____
_____   _____
_____   _____
_____   _____
_____   _____

MAINTENANCE / UPKEEP

SNIFF TEST: DRY CLEANERS? CHECK SHOES?

DAMAGE/REPAIRS NEEDED   (PUT IN SPECIAL PLACE)

_____   _____
_____   _____
_____   _____
_____   _____
_____   _____

END OF DAY OUTFIT REVIEW

HOW DID YOU FEEL? DID YOU GET COMPLIMENTS?
DID YOU REACH YOUR GOAL TODAY?

_____
_____
_____
_____
_____
_____
_____

DATE: _____ **DAY:** M T W TH F SAT SUN

YOUR MOOD: _____

WHO IS YOUR AUDIENCE?   (CIRCLE)

SHOPPING/ERRANDS   DOCTORS (SELF/KIDS)   TRAVEL

KIDS EVENTS   FAMILY FUNCTION   SINGLES EVENT

PROF. MEETINGS   CASUAL WORK DAY   HOME OFFICE DAY

FACE/FACE MEETING   ON-SITE CLIENT MEETING

NETWORKING   VIDEO CONFERENCE   PRESENTATION

DATE NIGHT   PARTY: CASUAL OR DRESSY   GIRLS NIGHT

HOLIDAY /SPECIAL EVENT   _____

_____   _____   _____

WHAT GOAL / MESSAGE ARE YOU COMMUNICATING ?
(BUSINESS AND OR PERSONAL)

BUILDING RAPPORT / TRUST   CONFIDENT / SELF-ASSURED

LEADER   INDEPENDENT / SELF-SUFFICIENT

FASCINATING / INTRIGING   EDUCATE / TEACH

CHARMING / ENGAGING   ALLURING / ROMANTIC

WEATHER:

RAIN   SNOW   SUNNY   HOT   HUMID

SPRING COLD/WARM   SUMMER COOL/HOT   FALL COLD/WARM

WINTER COLD/WARM   UMBRELLA   RAINCOAT

BACK UP SHOES   BOOTS / TRACK SHOES   _____

WHICH STYLE WORDS ARE YOU COMMUNICATING?

CONFIDENT   PROFESSIONAL POWERFUL   SEXY   FUN

SAVVY   FRESH   MODERN   APPROACHABLE   AGELESS

PUT-TOGETHER   TRENDY   IN-CONTROL   WHIMSICAL

_____   _____   _____

MAIN WARDROBE EVENT: _____

TODAY'S OUTFIT   (REFER TO LOOK BOOK)

_____   _____
_____   _____
_____   _____
_____   _____
_____   _____
_____   _____
_____   _____
_____   _____

MAINTENANCE / UPKEEP

SNIFF TEST: DRY CLEANERS? CHECK SHOES?

DAMAGE/REPAIRS NEEDED   (PUT IN SPECIAL PLACE)

_____   _____
_____   _____
_____   _____
_____   _____
_____   _____

END OF DAY OUTFIT REVIEW

HOW DID YOU FEEL? DID YOU GET COMPLIMENTS?
DID YOU REACH YOUR GOAL TODAY?

_____
_____
_____
_____
_____
_____

If your jewelry is all boxed up in little boxes and stored in a drawer you're never going to wear it. You need to see it to use it.

Let them come out and play!

The

LOOK BOOK

is the secret

sauce to your

success!!

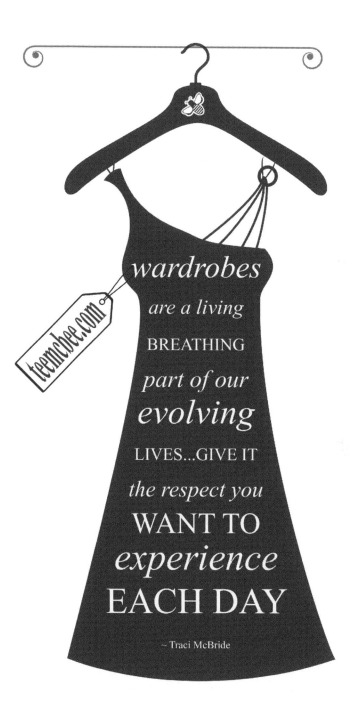

teemcbee.com

wardrobes *are a living* BREATHING *part of our* *evolving* LIVES...GIVE IT *the respect you* WANT TO *experience* EACH DAY

~ Traci McBride

DATE: _____ **DAY:** M T W TH F SAT SUN

YOUR MOOD: _____

WHO IS YOUR AUDIENCE? (CIRCLE)

SHOPPING/ERRANDS   DOCTORS (SELF/KIDS)   TRAVEL

KIDS EVENTS   FAMILY FUNCTION   SINGLES EVENT

PROF. MEETINGS   CASUAL WORK DAY   HOME OFFICE DAY

FACE/FACE MEETING   ON-SITE CLIENT MEETING

NETWORKING   VIDEO CONFERENCE   PRESENTATION

DATE NIGHT   PARTY: CASUAL OR DRESSY   GIRLS NIGHT

HOLIDAY /SPECIAL EVENT   _____

_____   _____   _____

WHAT GOAL / MESSAGE ARE YOU COMMUNICATING ?
(BUSINESS AND OR PERSONAL)

BUILDING RAPPORT / TRUST   CONFIDENT / SELF-ASSURED

LEADER   INDEPENDENT / SELF-SUFFICIENT

FASCINATING / INTRIGING   EDUCATE / TEACH

CHARMING / ENGAGING   ALLURING / ROMANTIC

WEATHER:

RAIN   SNOW   SUNNY   HOT   HUMID

SPRING COLD/WARM   SUMMER COOL/HOT   FALL COLD/WARM

WINTER COLD/WARM   UMBRELLA   RAINCOAT

BACK UP SHOES   BOOTS / TRACK SHOES   _____

WHICH STYLE WORDS ARE YOU COMMUNICATING?

CONFIDENT   PROFESSIONAL   POWERFUL   SEXY   FUN

SAVVY   FRESH   MODERN   APPROACHABLE   AGELESS

PUT-TOGETHER   TRENDY   IN-CONTROL   WHIMSICAL

_____   _____   _____

MAIN WARDROBE EVENT: _____

TODAY'S OUTFIT   (REFER TO LOOK BOOK)

_____   _____

_____   _____

_____   _____

_____   _____

_____   _____

_____   _____

_____   _____

MAINTENANCE / UPKEEP

SNIFF TEST: DRY CLEANERS? CHECK SHOES?

DAMAGE/REPAIRS NEEDED   (PUT IN SPECIAL PLACE)

_____   _____

_____   _____

_____   _____

_____   _____

END OF DAY OUTFIT REVIEW

HOW DID YOU FEEL? DID YOU GET COMPLIMENTS?
DID YOU REACH YOUR GOAL TODAY?

_____

_____

_____

_____

_____

_____

DATE: _____ **DAY:** M T W TH F SAT SUN

YOUR MOOD: _____

WHO IS YOUR AUDIENCE? (CIRCLE)

SHOPPING/ERRANDS   DOCTORS (SELF/KIDS)   TRAVEL

KIDS EVENTS   FAMILY FUNCTION   SINGLES EVENT

PROF. MEETINGS   CASUAL WORK DAY   HOME OFFICE DAY

FACE/FACE MEETING   ON-SITE CLIENT MEETING

NETWORKING   VIDEO CONFERENCE   PRESENTATION

DATE NIGHT   PARTY: CASUAL OR DRESSY   GIRLS NIGHT

HOLIDAY /SPECIAL EVENT   _____

_____   _____   _____

WHAT GOAL / MESSAGE ARE YOU COMMUNICATING ?
(BUSINESS AND OR PERSONAL)

BUILDING RAPPORT / TRUST   CONFIDENT / SELF-ASSURED

LEADER   INDEPENDENT / SELF-SUFFICIENT

FASCINATING / INTRIGING   EDUCATE / TEACH

CHARMING / ENGAGING   ALLURING / ROMANTIC

WEATHER:

RAIN   SNOW   SUNNY   HOT   HUMID

SPRING COLD/WARM   SUMMER COOL/HOT   FALL COLD/WARM

WINTER COLD/WARM   UMBRELLA   RAINCOAT

BACK UP SHOES   BOOTS / TRACK SHOES   _____

WHICH STYLE WORDS ARE YOU COMMUNICATING?

CONFIDENT   PROFESSIONAL   POWERFUL   SEXY   FUN

SAVVY   FRESH   MODERN   APPROACHABLE   AGELESS

PUT-TOGETHER   TRENDY   IN-CONTROL   WHIMSICAL

_____   _____   _____

MAIN WARDROBE EVENT: _____

TODAY'S OUTFIT   (REFER TO LOOK BOOK)

_____   _____
_____   _____
_____   _____
_____   _____
_____   _____
_____   _____
_____   _____

MAINTENANCE / UPKEEP

SNIFF TEST: DRY CLEANERS? CHECK SHOES?

DAMAGE/REPAIRS NEEDED   (PUT IN SPECIAL PLACE)

_____   _____
_____   _____
_____   _____
_____   _____
_____   _____

END OF DAY OUTFIT REVIEW

HOW DID YOU FEEL? DID YOU GET COMPLIMENTS?
DID YOU REACH YOUR GOAL TODAY?

_____
_____
_____
_____
_____
_____
_____

DATE: _____ **DAY:** M T W TH F SAT SUN

YOUR MOOD: _____

WHO IS YOUR AUDIENCE? (CIRCLE)

SHOPPING/ERRANDS   DOCTORS (SELF/KIDS)   TRAVEL

KIDS EVENTS   FAMILY FUNCTION   SINGLES EVENT

PROF. MEETINGS   CASUAL WORK DAY   HOME OFFICE DAY

FACE/FACE MEETING   ON-SITE CLIENT MEETING

NETWORKING   VIDEO CONFERENCE   PRESENTATION

DATE NIGHT   PARTY: CASUAL OR DRESSY   GIRLS NIGHT

HOLIDAY /SPECIAL EVENT   _____

_____   _____   _____

WHAT GOAL / MESSAGE ARE YOU COMMUNICATING ?
(BUSINESS AND OR PERSONAL)

BUILDING RAPPORT / TRUST   CONFIDENT / SELF-ASSURED

LEADER   INDEPENDENT / SELF-SUFFICIENT

FASCINATING / INTRIGING   EDUCATE / TEACH

CHARMING / ENGAGING   ALLURING / ROMANTIC

WEATHER:

RAIN   SNOW   SUNNY   HOT   HUMID

SPRING COLD/WARM   SUMMER COOL/HOT   FALL COLD/WARM

WINTER COLD/WARM   UMBRELLA   RAINCOAT

BACK UP SHOES   BOOTS / TRACK SHOES   _____

WHICH STYLE WORDS ARE YOU COMMUNICATING?

CONFIDENT   PROFESSIONAL   POWERFUL   SEXY   FUN

SAVVY   FRESH   MODERN   APPROACHABLE   AGELESS

PUT-TOGETHER   TRENDY   IN-CONTROL   WHIMSICAL

_____   _____   _____

MAIN WARDROBE EVENT: _____

TODAY'S OUTFIT   (REFER TO LOOK BOOK)

_____   _____
_____   _____
_____   _____
_____   _____
_____   _____
_____   _____
_____   _____

MAINTENANCE / UPKEEP

SNIFF TEST: DRY CLEANERS? CHECK SHOES?

DAMAGE/REPAIRS NEEDED   (PUT IN SPECIAL PLACE)

_____   _____
_____   _____
_____   _____
_____   _____

END OF DAY OUTFIT REVIEW

HOW DID YOU FEEL? DID YOU GET COMPLIMENTS?
DID YOU REACH YOUR GOAL TODAY?

_____
_____
_____
_____
_____
_____

DATE: _____ **DAY:** M T W TH F SAT SUN

YOUR MOOD: _____

WHO IS YOUR AUDIENCE?   (CIRCLE)

SHOPPING/ERRANDS   DOCTORS (SELF/KIDS)   TRAVEL

KIDS EVENTS   FAMILY FUNCTION   SINGLES EVENT

PROF. MEETINGS   CASUAL WORK DAY   HOME OFFICE DAY

FACE/FACE MEETING   ON-SITE CLIENT MEETING

NETWORKING   VIDEO CONFERENCE   PRESENTATION

DATE NIGHT   PARTY: CASUAL OR DRESSY   GIRLS NIGHT

HOLIDAY /SPECIAL EVENT   _____

_____   _____   _____

WHAT GOAL / MESSAGE ARE YOU COMMUNICATING ?
(BUSINESS AND OR PERSONAL)

BUILDING RAPPORT / TRUST   CONFIDENT / SELF-ASSURED

LEADER   INDEPENDENT / SELF-SUFFICIENT

FASCINATING / INTRIGING   EDUCATE / TEACH

CHARMING / ENGAGING   ALLURING / ROMANTIC

WEATHER:

RAIN   SNOW   SUNNY   HOT   HUMID

SPRING COLD/WARM   SUMMER COOL/HOT   FALL COLD/WARM

WINTER COLD/WARM   UMBRELLA   RAINCOAT

BACK UP SHOES   BOOTS / TRACK SHOES   _____

WHICH STYLE WORDS ARE YOU COMMUNICATING?

CONFIDENT   PROFESSIONAL   POWERFUL   SEXY   FUN

SAVVY   FRESH   MODERN   APPROACHABLE   AGELESS

PUT-TOGETHER   TRENDY   IN-CONTROL   WHIMSICAL

_____   _____   _____

MAIN WARDROBE EVENT: _____

TODAY'S OUTFIT   (REFER TO LOOK BOOK)

_____   _____
_____   _____
_____   _____
_____   _____
_____   _____
_____   _____
_____   _____

MAINTENANCE / UPKEEP

SNIFF TEST: DRY CLEANERS? CHECK SHOES?

DAMAGE/REPAIRS NEEDED   (PUT IN SPECIAL PLACE)

_____   _____
_____   _____
_____   _____
_____   _____

END OF DAY OUTFIT REVIEW

HOW DID YOU FEEL? DID YOU GET COMPLIMENTS?
DID YOU REACH YOUR GOAL TODAY?

_____
_____
_____
_____
_____
_____

Don't dry. Because drying your clothes is very hard on them and they will deteriorate quicker.

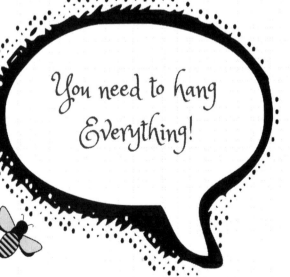

You need to hang Everything!

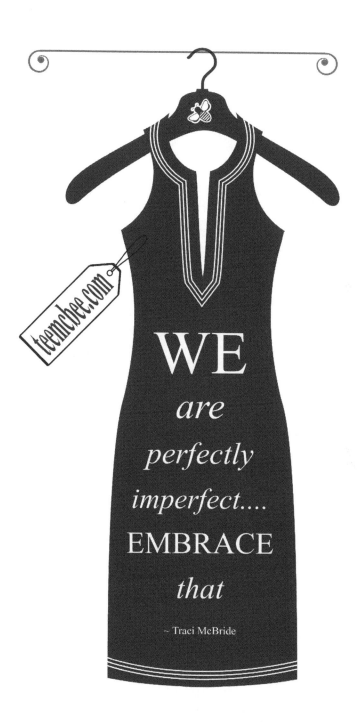

WE

are

perfectly

imperfect....

EMBRACE

that

~ Traci McBride

DATE: _____ **DAY:** M T W TH F SAT SUN

YOUR MOOD: _____

WHO IS YOUR AUDIENCE?   (CIRCLE)

SHOPPING/ERRANDS   DOCTORS (SELF/KIDS)   TRAVEL

KIDS EVENTS   FAMILY FUNCTION   SINGLES EVENT

PROF. MEETINGS   CASUAL WORK DAY   HOME OFFICE DAY

FACE/FACE MEETING   ON-SITE CLIENT MEETING

NETWORKING   VIDEO CONFERENCE   PRESENTATION

DATE NIGHT   PARTY: CASUAL OR DRESSY   GIRLS NIGHT

HOLIDAY /SPECIAL EVENT   _____

_____   _____   _____

WHAT GOAL / MESSAGE ARE YOU COMMUNICATING ?
(BUSINESS AND OR PERSONAL)

BUILDING RAPPORT / TRUST   CONFIDENT / SELF-ASSURED

LEADER   INDEPENDENT / SELF-SUFFICIENT

FASCINATING / INTRIGING   EDUCATE / TEACH

CHARMING / ENGAGING   ALLURING / ROMANTIC

WEATHER:

RAIN   SNOW   SUNNY   HOT   HUMID

SPRING COLD/WARM   SUMMER COOL/HOT   FALL COLD/WARM

WINTER COLD/WARM   UMBRELLA   RAINCOAT

BACK UP SHOES   BOOTS / TRACK SHOES   _____

WHICH STYLE WORDS ARE YOU COMMUNICATING?

CONFIDENT   PROFESSIONAL POWERFUL   SEXY   FUN

SAVVY   FRESH   MODERN   APPROACHABLE   AGELESS

PUT-TOGETHER   TRENDY   IN-CONTROL   WHIMSICAL

_____   _____   _____

MAIN WARDROBE EVENT: _____

TODAY'S OUTFIT   (REFER TO LOOK BOOK)

_____   _____
_____   _____
_____   _____
_____   _____
_____   _____
_____   _____
_____   _____
_____   _____

MAINTENANCE / UPKEEP

SNIFF TEST: DRY CLEANERS? CHECK SHOES?

DAMAGE/REPAIRS NEEDED   (PUT IN SPECIAL PLACE)

_____   _____
_____   _____
_____   _____
_____   _____
_____   _____

END OF DAY OUTFIT REVIEW

HOW DID YOU FEEL? DID YOU GET COMPLIMENTS?
DID YOU REACH YOUR GOAL TODAY?

_____
_____
_____
_____
_____
_____

DATE: _____ **DAY:** M T W TH F SAT SUN

YOUR MOOD: _____

WHO IS YOUR AUDIENCE? (CIRCLE)

SHOPPING/ERRANDS   DOCTORS (SELF/KIDS)   TRAVEL

KIDS EVENTS   FAMILY FUNCTION   SINGLES EVENT

PROF. MEETINGS   CASUAL WORK DAY   HOME OFFICE DAY

FACE/FACE MEETING   ON-SITE CLIENT MEETING

NETWORKING   VIDEO CONFERENCE   PRESENTATION

DATE NIGHT   PARTY: CASUAL OR DRESSY   GIRLS NIGHT

HOLIDAY /SPECIAL EVENT   _____

_____   _____   _____

WHAT GOAL / MESSAGE ARE YOU COMMUNICATING ?
(BUSINESS AND OR PERSONAL)

BUILDING RAPPORT / TRUST   CONFIDENT / SELF-ASSURED

LEADER   INDEPENDENT / SELF-SUFFICIENT

FASCINATING / INTRIGING   EDUCATE / TEACH

CHARMING / ENGAGING   ALLURING / ROMANTIC

WEATHER:

RAIN   SNOW   SUNNY   HOT   HUMID

SPRING COLD/WARM   SUMMER COOL/HOT   FALL COLD/WARM

WINTER COLD/WARM   UMBRELLA   RAINCOAT

BACK UP SHOES   BOOTS / TRACK SHOES   _____

WHICH STYLE WORDS ARE YOU COMMUNICATING?

CONFIDENT   PROFESSIONAL   POWERFUL   SEXY   FUN

SAVVY   FRESH   MODERN   APPROACHABLE   AGELESS

PUT-TOGETHER   TRENDY   IN-CONTROL   WHIMSICAL

_____   _____   _____

MAIN WARDROBE EVENT: _____

TODAY'S OUTFIT   (REFER TO LOOK BOOK)

_____   _____
_____   _____
_____   _____
_____   _____
_____   _____
_____   _____
_____   _____

MAINTENANCE / UPKEEP

SNIFF TEST: DRY CLEANERS? CHECK SHOES?

DAMAGE/REPAIRS NEEDED   (PUT IN SPECIAL PLACE)

_____   _____
_____   _____
_____   _____
_____   _____
_____   _____

END OF DAY OUTFIT REVIEW

HOW DID YOU FEEL? DID YOU GET COMPLIMENTS?
DID YOU REACH YOUR GOAL TODAY?

_____
_____
_____
_____
_____
_____

DATE: _____ DAY: M T W   TH   F   SAT   SUN

YOUR MOOD: _____

WHO IS YOUR AUDIENCE? (CIRCLE)

SHOPPING/ERRANDS   DOCTORS (SELF/KIDS)   TRAVEL

KIDS EVENTS   FAMILY FUNCTION   SINGLES EVENT

PROF. MEETINGS   CASUAL WORK DAY   HOME OFFICE DAY

FACE/FACE MEETING   ON-SITE CLIENT MEETING

NETWORKING   VIDEO CONFERENCE   PRESENTATION

DATE NIGHT   PARTY: CASUAL OR DRESSY   GIRLS NIGHT

HOLIDAY /SPECIAL EVENT   _____

_____   _____   _____

WHAT GOAL / MESSAGE ARE YOU COMMUNICATING ?
(BUSINESS AND OR PERSONAL)

BUILDING RAPPORT / TRUST   CONFIDENT / SELF-ASSURED

LEADER   INDEPENDENT / SELF-SUFFICIENT

FASCINATING / INTRIGING   EDUCATE / TEACH

CHARMING / ENGAGING   ALLURING / ROMANTIC

WEATHER:

RAIN   SNOW   SUNNY   HOT   HUMID

SPRING COLD/WARM   SUMMER COOL/HOT   FALL COLD/WARM

WINTER COLD/WARM   UMBRELLA   RAINCOAT

BACK UP SHOES   BOOTS / TRACK SHOES   _____

WHICH STYLE WORDS ARE YOU COMMUNICATING?

CONFIDENT   PROFESSIONAL POWERFUL   SEXY   FUN

SAVVY   FRESH   MODERN   APPROACHABLE   AGELESS

PUT-TOGETHER   TRENDY   IN-CONTROL   WHIMSICAL

_____   _____   _____

MAIN WARDROBE EVENT: _____

TODAY'S OUTFIT   (REFER TO LOOK BOOK)

_____   _____
_____   _____
_____   _____
_____   _____
_____   _____
_____   _____
_____   _____

MAINTENANCE / UPKEEP

SNIFF TEST: DRY CLEANERS? CHECK SHOES?

DAMAGE/REPAIRS NEEDED   (PUT IN SPECIAL PLACE)

_____   _____
_____   _____
_____   _____
_____   _____

END OF DAY OUTFIT REVIEW

HOW DID YOU FEEL? DID YOU GET COMPLIMENTS?
DID YOU REACH YOUR GOAL TODAY?

_____
_____
_____
_____
_____
_____

DATE: _____ DAY: M T W TH F SAT SUN

YOUR MOOD: _____

WHO IS YOUR AUDIENCE? (CIRCLE)

SHOPPING/ERRANDS DOCTORS (SELF/KIDS) TRAVEL

KIDS EVENTS FAMILY FUNCTION SINGLES EVENT

PROF. MEETINGS CASUAL WORK DAY HOME OFFICE DAY

FACE/FACE MEETING ON-SITE CLIENT MEETING

NETWORKING VIDEO CONFERENCE PRESENTATION

DATE NIGHT PARTY: CASUAL OR DRESSY GIRLS NIGHT

HOLIDAY /SPECIAL EVENT _____

_____ _____ _____

WHAT GOAL / MESSAGE ARE YOU COMMUNICATING ?
(BUSINESS AND OR PERSONAL)

BUILDING RAPPORT / TRUST CONFIDENT / SELF-ASSURED

LEADER INDEPENDENT / SELF-SUFFICIENT

FASCINATING / INTRIGING EDUCATE / TEACH

CHARMING / ENGAGING ALLURING / ROMANTIC

WEATHER:

RAIN SNOW SUNNY HOT HUMID

SPRING COLD/WARM SUMMER COOL/HOT FALL COLD/WARM

WINTER COLD/WARM UMBRELLA RAINCOAT

BACK UP SHOES BOOTS / TRACK SHOES _____

WHICH STYLE WORDS ARE YOU COMMUNICATING?

CONFIDENT PROFESSIONAL POWERFUL SEXY FUN

SAVVY FRESH MODERN APPROACHABLE AGELESS

PUT-TOGETHER TRENDY IN-CONTROL WHIMSICAL

_____ _____ _____

MAIN WARDROBE EVENT: _____

TODAY'S OUTFIT   (REFER TO LOOK BOOK)

_____   _____
_____   _____
_____   _____
_____   _____
_____   _____
_____   _____
_____   _____
_____   _____

MAINTENANCE / UPKEEP

SNIFF TEST: DRY CLEANERS? CHECK SHOES?

DAMAGE/REPAIRS NEEDED   (PUT IN SPECIAL PLACE)

_____   _____
_____   _____
_____   _____
_____   _____
_____   _____

END OF DAY OUTFIT REVIEW

HOW DID YOU FEEL? DID YOU GET COMPLIMENTS?
DID YOU REACH YOUR GOAL TODAY?

_____
_____
_____
_____
_____
_____
_____

DATE: _____ **DAY:** M T W TH F SAT SUN

YOUR MOOD: _____

WHO IS YOUR AUDIENCE? (CIRCLE)

SHOPPING/ERRANDS   DOCTORS (SELF/KIDS)   TRAVEL

KIDS EVENTS   FAMILY FUNCTION   SINGLES EVENT

PROF. MEETINGS   CASUAL WORK DAY   HOME OFFICE DAY

FACE/FACE MEETING   ON-SITE CLIENT MEETING

NETWORKING   VIDEO CONFERENCE   PRESENTATION

DATE NIGHT   PARTY: CASUAL OR DRESSY   GIRLS NIGHT

HOLIDAY /SPECIAL EVENT   _____

_____   _____   _____

WHAT GOAL / MESSAGE ARE YOU COMMUNICATING ?
(BUSINESS AND OR PERSONAL)

BUILDING RAPPORT / TRUST   CONFIDENT / SELF-ASSURED

LEADER   INDEPENDENT / SELF-SUFFICIENT

FASCINATING / INTRIGING   EDUCATE / TEACH

CHARMING / ENGAGING   ALLURING / ROMANTIC

WEATHER:

RAIN   SNOW   SUNNY   HOT   HUMID

SPRING COLD/WARM   SUMMER COOL/HOT   FALL COLD/WARM

WINTER COLD/WARM   UMBRELLA   RAINCOAT

BACK UP SHOES   BOOTS / TRACK SHOES   _____

WHICH STYLE WORDS ARE YOU COMMUNICATING?

CONFIDENT   PROFESSIONAL POWERFUL   SEXY   FUN

SAVVY   FRESH   MODERN   APPROACHABLE   AGELESS

PUT-TOGETHER   TRENDY   IN-CONTROL   WHIMSICAL

_____   _____   _____

MAIN WARDROBE EVENT: _____

TODAY'S OUTFIT   (REFER TO LOOK BOOK)

_____   _____
_____   _____
_____   _____
_____   _____
_____   _____
_____   _____
_____   _____

MAINTENANCE / UPKEEP

SNIFF TEST: DRY CLEANERS? CHECK SHOES?

DAMAGE/REPAIRS NEEDED   (PUT IN SPECIAL PLACE)

_____   _____
_____   _____
_____   _____
_____   _____

END OF DAY OUTFIT REVIEW

HOW DID YOU FEEL? DID YOU GET COMPLIMENTS?
DID YOU REACH YOUR GOAL TODAY?

_____
_____
_____
_____
_____
_____
_____

DATE: _____ **DAY:** M T W TH F SAT SUN

YOUR MOOD: _____

WHO IS YOUR AUDIENCE? (CIRCLE)

SHOPPING/ERRANDS   DOCTORS (SELF/KIDS)   TRAVEL

KIDS EVENTS   FAMILY FUNCTION   SINGLES EVENT

PROF. MEETINGS   CASUAL WORK DAY   HOME OFFICE DAY

FACE/FACE MEETING   ON-SITE CLIENT MEETING

NETWORKING   VIDEO CONFERENCE   PRESENTATION

DATE NIGHT   PARTY: CASUAL OR DRESSY   GIRLS NIGHT

HOLIDAY /SPECIAL EVENT   _____

_____   _____   _____

WHAT GOAL / MESSAGE ARE YOU COMMUNICATING ?
(BUSINESS AND OR PERSONAL)

BUILDING RAPPORT / TRUST   CONFIDENT / SELF-ASSURED

LEADER   INDEPENDENT / SELF-SUFFICIENT

FASCINATING / INTRIGING   EDUCATE / TEACH

CHARMING / ENGAGING   ALLURING / ROMANTIC

WEATHER:

RAIN   SNOW   SUNNY   HOT   HUMID

SPRING COLD/WARM   SUMMER COOL/HOT   FALL COLD/WARM

WINTER COLD/WARM   UMBRELLA   RAINCOAT

BACK UP SHOES   BOOTS / TRACK SHOES   _____

WHICH STYLE WORDS ARE YOU COMMUNICATING?

CONFIDENT   PROFESSIONAL POWERFUL   SEXY   FUN

SAVVY   FRESH   MODERN   APPROACHABLE   AGELESS

PUT-TOGETHER   TRENDY   IN-CONTROL   WHIMSICAL

_____   _____   _____

MAIN WARDROBE EVENT: _____

TODAY'S OUTFIT   (REFER TO LOOK BOOK)

_____   _____

_____   _____

_____   _____

_____   _____

_____   _____

_____   _____

_____   _____

MAINTENANCE / UPKEEP

SNIFF TEST: DRY CLEANERS? CHECK SHOES?

DAMAGE/REPAIRS NEEDED   (PUT IN SPECIAL PLACE)

_____   _____

_____   _____

_____   _____

_____   _____

END OF DAY OUTFIT REVIEW

HOW DID YOU FEEL? DID YOU GET COMPLIMENTS?
DID YOU REACH YOUR GOAL TODAY?

_____

_____

_____

_____

_____

_____

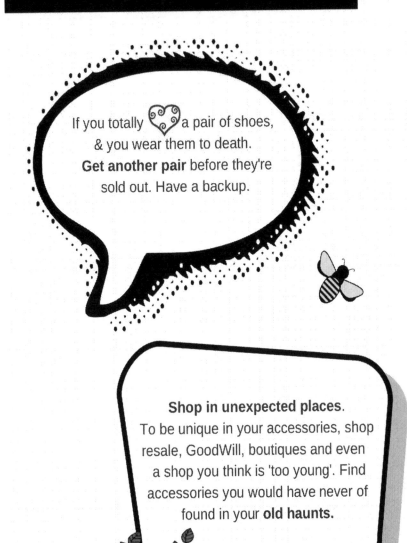

If you totally ♡ a pair of shoes,
& you wear them to death.
Get another pair before they're
sold out. Have a backup.

Shop in unexpected places.
To be unique in your accessories, shop
resale, GoodWill, boutiques and even
a shop you think is 'too young'. Find
accessories you would have never of
found in your **old haunts.**

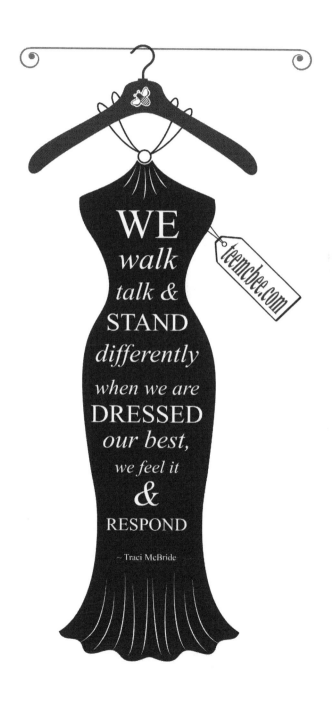

WE *walk talk* & STAND *differently when we are* DRESSED *our best, we feel it* & RESPOND

~ Traci McBride

teemcbee.com

DATE: _____ **DAY:** M T W TH F SAT SUN

YOUR MOOD: _____

WHO IS YOUR AUDIENCE?   (CIRCLE)

SHOPPING/ERRANDS   DOCTORS (SELF/KIDS)   TRAVEL

KIDS EVENTS   FAMILY FUNCTION   SINGLES EVENT

PROF. MEETINGS   CASUAL WORK DAY   HOME OFFICE DAY

FACE/FACE MEETING   ON-SITE CLIENT MEETING

NETWORKING   VIDEO CONFERENCE   PRESENTATION

DATE NIGHT   PARTY: CASUAL OR DRESSY   GIRLS NIGHT

HOLIDAY /SPECIAL EVENT   _____

_____   _____   _____

WHAT GOAL / MESSAGE ARE YOU COMMUNICATING ?
(BUSINESS AND OR PERSONAL)

BUILDING RAPPORT / TRUST   CONFIDENT / SELF-ASSURED

LEADER   INDEPENDENT / SELF-SUFFICIENT

FASCINATING / INTRIGING   EDUCATE / TEACH

CHARMING / ENGAGING   ALLURING / ROMANTIC

WEATHER:

RAIN   SNOW   SUNNY   HOT   HUMID

SPRING COLD/WARM   SUMMER COOL/HOT   FALL COLD/WARM

WINTER COLD/WARM   UMBRELLA   RAINCOAT

BACK UP SHOES   BOOTS / TRACK SHOES   _____

WHICH STYLE WORDS ARE YOU COMMUNICATING?

CONFIDENT   PROFESSIONAL   POWERFUL   SEXY   FUN

SAVVY   FRESH   MODERN   APPROACHABLE   AGELESS

PUT-TOGETHER   TRENDY   IN-CONTROL   WHIMSICAL

_____   _____   _____

MAIN WARDROBE EVENT: _____

TODAY'S OUTFIT   (REFER TO LOOK BOOK)

_____   _____
_____   _____
_____   _____
_____   _____
_____   _____
_____   _____
_____   _____

MAINTENANCE / UPKEEP

SNIFF TEST: DRY CLEANERS? CHECK SHOES?

DAMAGE/REPAIRS NEEDED   (PUT IN SPECIAL PLACE)

_____   _____
_____   _____
_____   _____
_____   _____

END OF DAY OUTFIT REVIEW

HOW DID YOU FEEL? DID YOU GET COMPLIMENTS?
DID YOU REACH YOUR GOAL TODAY?

_____
_____
_____
_____
_____
_____

DATE: _____ DAY: M T W TH F SAT SUN

YOUR MOOD: _____

WHO IS YOUR AUDIENCE?   (CIRCLE)

SHOPPING/ERRANDS   DOCTORS (SELF/KIDS)   TRAVEL

KIDS EVENTS   FAMILY FUNCTION   SINGLES EVENT

PROF. MEETINGS   CASUAL WORK DAY   HOME OFFICE DAY

FACE/FACE MEETING   ON-SITE CLIENT MEETING

NETWORKING   VIDEO CONFERENCE   PRESENTATION

DATE NIGHT   PARTY: CASUAL OR DRESSY   GIRLS NIGHT

HOLIDAY /SPECIAL EVENT   _____

_____   _____   _____

WHAT GOAL / MESSAGE ARE YOU COMMUNICATING ?
(BUSINESS AND OR PERSONAL)

BUILDING RAPPORT / TRUST   CONFIDENT / SELF-ASSURED

LEADER   INDEPENDENT / SELF-SUFFICIENT

FASCINATING / INTRIGING   EDUCATE / TEACH

CHARMING / ENGAGING   ALLURING / ROMANTIC

WEATHER:

RAIN   SNOW   SUNNY   HOT   HUMID

SPRING COLD/WARM   SUMMER COOL/HOT   FALL COLD/WARM

WINTER COLD/WARM   UMBRELLA   RAINCOAT

BACK UP SHOES   BOOTS / TRACK SHOES   _____

WHICH STYLE WORDS ARE YOU COMMUNICATING?

CONFIDENT   PROFESSIONAL POWERFUL   SEXY   FUN

SAVVY   FRESH   MODERN   APPROACHABLE   AGELESS

PUT-TOGETHER   TRENDY   IN-CONTROL   WHIMSICAL

_____   _____   _____

MAIN WARDROBE EVENT: _____

TODAY'S OUTFIT   (REFER TO LOOK BOOK)

_____   _____
_____   _____
_____   _____
_____   _____
_____   _____
_____   _____
_____   _____

MAINTENANCE / UPKEEP

SNIFF TEST: DRY CLEANERS? CHECK SHOES?

DAMAGE/REPAIRS NEEDED   (PUT IN SPECIAL PLACE)

_____   _____
_____   _____
_____   _____
_____   _____

END OF DAY OUTFIT REVIEW

HOW DID YOU FEEL? DID YOU GET COMPLIMENTS?
DID YOU REACH YOUR GOAL TODAY?

_____
_____
_____
_____
_____
_____

DATE: _____ **DAY:** M T W TH F SAT SUN

YOUR MOOD: _____

WHO IS YOUR AUDIENCE?   (CIRCLE)

SHOPPING/ERRANDS   DOCTORS (SELF/KIDS)   TRAVEL

KIDS EVENTS   FAMILY FUNCTION   SINGLES EVENT

PROF. MEETINGS   CASUAL WORK DAY   HOME OFFICE DAY

FACE/FACE MEETING   ON-SITE CLIENT MEETING

NETWORKING   VIDEO CONFERENCE   PRESENTATION

DATE NIGHT   PARTY: CASUAL OR DRESSY   GIRLS NIGHT

HOLIDAY /SPECIAL EVENT   _____

_____   _____   _____

WHAT GOAL / MESSAGE ARE YOU COMMUNICATING ?
(BUSINESS AND OR PERSONAL)

BUILDING RAPPORT / TRUST   CONFIDENT / SELF-ASSURED

LEADER   INDEPENDENT / SELF-SUFFICIENT

FASCINATING / INTRIGING   EDUCATE / TEACH

CHARMING / ENGAGING   ALLURING / ROMANTIC

WEATHER:

RAIN   SNOW   SUNNY   HOT   HUMID

SPRING COLD/WARM   SUMMER COOL/HOT   FALL COLD/WARM

WINTER COLD/WARM   UMBRELLA   RAINCOAT

BACK UP SHOES   BOOTS / TRACK SHOES   _____

WHICH STYLE WORDS ARE YOU COMMUNICATING?

CONFIDENT   PROFESSIONAL POWERFUL   SEXY   FUN

SAVVY   FRESH   MODERN   APPROACHABLE   AGELESS

PUT-TOGETHER   TRENDY   IN-CONTROL   WHIMSICAL

_____   _____   _____

MAIN WARDROBE EVENT: _____

TODAY'S OUTFIT   (REFER TO LOOK BOOK)

MAINTENANCE / UPKEEP

SNIFF TEST: DRY CLEANERS? CHECK SHOES?

DAMAGE/REPAIRS NEEDED   (PUT IN SPECIAL PLACE)

END OF DAY OUTFIT REVIEW

HOW DID YOU FEEL? DID YOU GET COMPLIMENTS?
DID YOU REACH YOUR GOAL TODAY?

DATE: _____ DAY: M T W TH F SAT SUN

YOUR MOOD: _____

WHO IS YOUR AUDIENCE?   (CIRCLE)

SHOPPING/ERRANDS   DOCTORS (SELF/KIDS)   TRAVEL

KIDS EVENTS   FAMILY FUNCTION   SINGLES EVENT

PROF. MEETINGS   CASUAL WORK DAY   HOME OFFICE DAY

FACE/FACE MEETING   ON-SITE CLIENT MEETING

NETWORKING   VIDEO CONFERENCE   PRESENTATION

DATE NIGHT   PARTY: CASUAL OR DRESSY   GIRLS NIGHT

HOLIDAY /SPECIAL EVENT   _____

_____   _____   _____

WHAT GOAL / MESSAGE ARE YOU COMMUNICATING?
(BUSINESS AND OR PERSONAL)

BUILDING RAPPORT / TRUST   CONFIDENT / SELF-ASSURED

LEADER   INDEPENDENT / SELF-SUFFICIENT

FASCINATING / INTRIGING   EDUCATE / TEACH

CHARMING / ENGAGING   ALLURING / ROMANTIC

WEATHER:

RAIN   SNOW   SUNNY   HOT   HUMID

SPRING COLD/WARM   SUMMER COOL/HOT   FALL COLD/WARM

WINTER COLD/WARM   UMBRELLA   RAINCOAT

BACK UP SHOES   BOOTS / TRACK SHOES   _____

WHICH STYLE WORDS ARE YOU COMMUNICATING?

CONFIDENT   PROFESSIONAL POWERFUL   SEXY   FUN

SAVVY   FRESH   MODERN   APPROACHABLE   AGELESS

PUT-TOGETHER   TRENDY   IN-CONTROL   WHIMSICAL

_____   _____   _____

MAIN WARDROBE EVENT: _____

TODAY'S OUTFIT   (REFER TO LOOK BOOK)

MAINTENANCE / UPKEEP

SNIFF TEST: DRY CLEANERS? CHECK SHOES?

DAMAGE/REPAIRS NEEDED   (PUT IN SPECIAL PLACE)

END OF DAY OUTFIT REVIEW

HOW DID YOU FEEL? DID YOU GET COMPLIMENTS?
DID YOU REACH YOUR GOAL TODAY?

Schedule at least 1 day a week for mending, cleaning, and pilling your wardrobe.

Your clothes will thank you, and so will your **wallet**.

MAKE YOUR MORNINGS EVEN EASIER– PULL YOUR OUTFITS FOR A FEW DAYS IN ADVANCE– OR EVEN A WEEK EARLY!

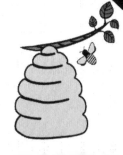

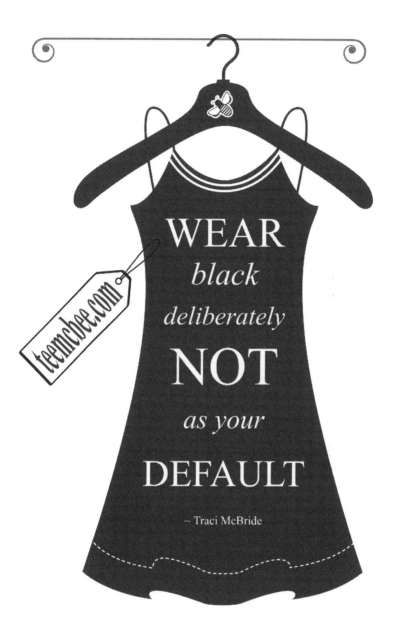

WEAR *black* *deliberately* NOT *as your* DEFAULT

~ Traci McBride

DATE: _____ DAY: M T W TH F SAT SUN

YOUR MOOD: _____

WHO IS YOUR AUDIENCE? (CIRCLE)

SHOPPING/ERRANDS   DOCTORS (SELF/KIDS)   TRAVEL

KIDS EVENTS   FAMILY FUNCTION   SINGLES EVENT

PROF. MEETINGS   CASUAL WORK DAY   HOME OFFICE DAY

FACE/FACE MEETING   ON-SITE CLIENT MEETING

NETWORKING   VIDEO CONFERENCE   PRESENTATION

DATE NIGHT   PARTY: CASUAL OR DRESSY   GIRLS NIGHT

HOLIDAY /SPECIAL EVENT   _____

_____   _____   _____

WHAT GOAL / MESSAGE ARE YOU COMMUNICATING ?
(BUSINESS AND OR PERSONAL)

BUILDING RAPPORT / TRUST   CONFIDENT / SELF-ASSURED

LEADER   INDEPENDENT / SELF-SUFFICIENT

FASCINATING / INTRIGING   EDUCATE / TEACH

CHARMING / ENGAGING   ALLURING / ROMANTIC

WEATHER:

RAIN   SNOW   SUNNY   HOT   HUMID

SPRING COLD/WARM   SUMMER COOL/HOT   FALL COLD/WARM

WINTER COLD/WARM   UMBRELLA   RAINCOAT

BACK UP SHOES   BOOTS / TRACK SHOES   _____

WHICH STYLE WORDS ARE YOU COMMUNICATING?

CONFIDENT   PROFESSIONAL POWERFUL   SEXY   FUN

SAVVY   FRESH   MODERN   APPROACHABLE   AGELESS

PUT-TOGETHER   TRENDY   IN-CONTROL   WHIMSICAL

_____   _____   _____

MAIN WARDROBE EVENT: _____

TODAY'S OUTFIT (REFER TO LOOK BOOK)

_____ _____
_____ _____
_____ _____
_____ _____
_____ _____
_____ _____
_____ _____

MAINTENANCE / UPKEEP

SNIFF TEST: DRY CLEANERS? CHECK SHOES?

DAMAGE/REPAIRS NEEDED   (PUT IN SPECIAL PLACE)

_____ _____
_____ _____
_____ _____
_____ _____
_____ _____

END OF DAY OUTFIT REVIEW

HOW DID YOU FEEL? DID YOU GET COMPLIMENTS?
DID YOU REACH YOUR GOAL TODAY?

_____
_____
_____
_____
_____
_____

DATE: _____ **DAY:** M T W TH F SAT SUN

 YOUR MOOD: _____

WHO IS YOUR AUDIENCE? (CIRCLE)

TRAVEL

SHOPPING/ERRANDS   DOCTORS (SELF/KIDS)

KIDS EVENTS   FAMILY FUNCTION   SINGLES EVENT

PROF. MEETINGS   CASUAL WORK DAY   HOME OFFICE DAY

FACE/FACE MEETING   ON-SITE CLIENT MEETING

NETWORKING   VIDEO CONFERENCE   PRESENTATION

DATE NIGHT   PARTY: CASUAL OR DRESSY   GIRLS NIGHT

HOLIDAY /SPECIAL EVENT   _____

_____   _____   _____

WHAT GOAL / MESSAGE ARE YOU COMMUNICATING?
(BUSINESS AND OR PERSONAL)

BUILDING RAPPORT / TRUST   CONFIDENT / SELF-ASSURED

LEADER   INDEPENDENT / SELF-SUFFICIENT

FASCINATING / INTRIGING   EDUCATE / TEACH

CHARMING / ENGAGING   ALLURING / ROMANTIC

WEATHER:

RAIN   SNOW   SUNNY   HOT   HUMID

SPRING COLD/WARM   SUMMER COOL/HOT   FALL COLD/WARM

WINTER COLD/WARM   UMBRELLA   RAINCOAT

BACK UP SHOES   BOOTS / TRACK SHOES   _____

WHICH STYLE WORDS ARE YOU COMMUNICATING?

CONFIDENT   PROFESSIONAL POWERFUL   SEXY   FUN

SAVVY   FRESH   MODERN   APPROACHABLE AGELESS

PUT-TOGETHER   TRENDY   IN-CONTROL   WHIMSICAL

_____   _____   _____

MAIN WARDROBE EVENT: _____

TODAY'S OUTFIT   (REFER TO LOOK BOOK)

_____   _____
_____   _____
_____   _____
_____   _____
_____   _____
_____   _____
_____   _____

MAINTENANCE / UPKEEP

SNIFF TEST: DRY CLEANERS? CHECK SHOES?

DAMAGE/REPAIRS NEEDED   (PUT IN SPECIAL PLACE)

_____   _____
_____   _____
_____   _____
_____   _____
_____   _____

END OF DAY OUTFIT REVIEW

HOW DID YOU FEEL? DID YOU GET COMPLIMENTS?
DID YOU REACH YOUR GOAL TODAY?

_____
_____
_____
_____
_____
_____

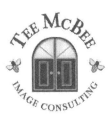

Congratulations
You completed your
first 30-day journal

Where do you go from here?
Return to the online book retailer and
purchase the book again.

OR

If you want just the log pages and nothing
else, we MIGHT be offering a
60-day log book, if there is enough interest.
Let us know if you are interested
in having this new book.
email: Traci@TeeMcBee.com

subject line: I WANT 60-DAY LOG!

NOTES & QUESTIONS

WRITE TO TRACI@TEEMCBEE.COM

_____
_____
_____
_____
_____
_____
_____
_____
_____
_____
_____
_____
_____
_____
_____
_____
_____

She could use your questions in her newsletter
or other social media Q&A's

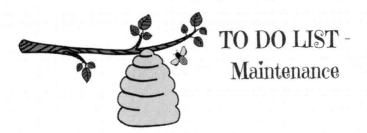

TO DO LIST -
Maintenance

_____

_____

_____

_____

_____

_____

_____

_____

_____

_____

_____

_____

_____

_____

_____

_____

_____

_____

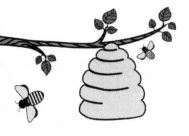

TO DO LIST
NOTES

_____

_____

_____

_____

_____

_____

_____

_____

_____

_____

_____

_____

_____

_____

_____

_____

_____

_____

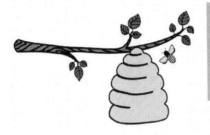

TEE'S
TOOL BOX

- ❦ VISIT TEEMCBEE'S PINTEREST BOARD

- ❦ BLOG ON TEEMCBEE.COM

- ❦ FRESH PERSPECTIVE NEWSLETTER-
  SIGN UP ON TEEMCBEE.COM

- ❦ LIKE TeeMcBee on FACEBOOK for more tips

- ❦ FOLLOW TeeMcBee on TWITTER

- ❦ FOLLOW TeeMcBee on INSTAGRAM

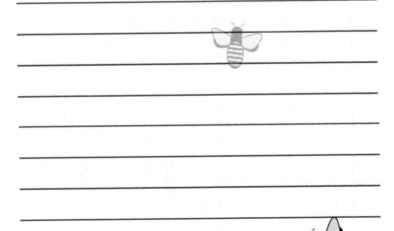

RESOURCES you found

Doodles of Inspiration

Doodles of Inspiration

A Little About Traci

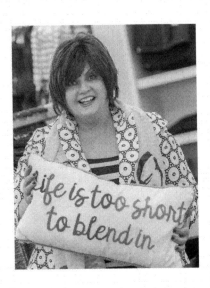

Traci McBride is the Chief Stylist with TeeMcBee Image Consulting, which specializes in elevating confidence & influence with your wardrobe. Traci provides wardrobe consultant's, **staff workshops** and **speaking on the topic of elevating personal brand** as well as **company branding**. Traci can be reached at **Traci@TeeMcBee.com**

Tee's Bio

Traci applies the knowledge and experience of her thirty plus year sales/marketing and fashion career along with her own life lessons to her current work of aiding people and businesses in polishing their most valuable asset – themselves.

Whether the client is a young professional developing her workplace image, a stay at home mother returning to the workforce or over 50 evolving and transitioning into the next stage of life. TeeMcBee customizes personal image services with sessions for **Closet Detox**, **Power Shopping**, **MASTER the MIXX**™ & **LOOK BOOK** photo shoots. Men and women can create the best version of themselves regardless of age, income, size or circumstance.

Traci will help identify habits or practices a client has developed that now sabotage their self-image and confidence. Once those habits are tamed, Traci will help translate the client's fresh perspective of self into a style and image to look forward to each morning.

Services
with Tee

#1 **closet detox** BY TEEMCBEE®

☐ Need to schedule
☐ Scheduled _____
☐ Need mini refreshener

#2 **POWER COLOR analysis** by TeeMcBee®

☐ Need to schedule
☐ Scheduled _____
☐ Gift 'Power of Color' for
   a friend

#3 **POWER shopping** with TeeMcBee®

☐ Need to schedule
☐ Schedule _____
☐ Need mini refreshener

#4 **MASTER the MIXX** with TeeMcBee®

☐ Need to schedule
☐ Schedule _____
☐ Need mini refreshener

Services with Tee

#5 LOOKbook *by TeeMcBee®*

- ☐ Need to schedule
- ☐ Scheduled _____
- ☐ Need mini refreshener

#6 *effortless* **PACKING** *with TeeMcBee®*

- ☐ Need to schedule
- ☐ Scheduled _____
- ☐ Need mini refreshener

#7 *Style* think TANK *by TeeMcBee*

Book an event for your Family/Friends

- ☐ Love to have a fun night- Need to schedule
- ☐ Scheduled _____

#8 TeeMcBee speaks

Speaker / Referral

Need a speaker?

- ☐ Give a Referral to an organization or event

Notes

Outside of Ohio but still want to work with Tee?

TEE WORKS VIRTUALLY!

(ZOOM, SKYPE, FACETIME, ETC.)

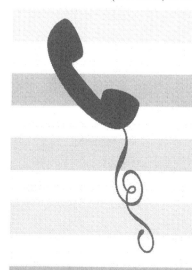

Or go to
goo.gl/KLmpum
(case sensitive)

Notes

SHARE THE LOVE

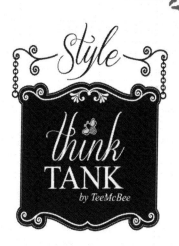

BOOK A SMALL GATHERING OF FRIENDS & FAMILY WHO LOVE TO TALK STYLE.

For details check out:

http://www.teemcbee.com/style-think-tank/

Notes

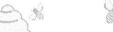

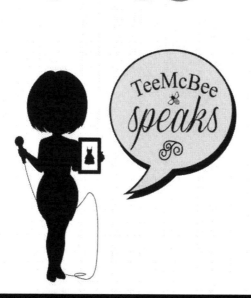

Notes

Bonus Tips by Tee

EFFORTLESS PACKING© TIPS & CHECKLIST

Effortless Packing Tips & Tidbits

This book is the best tool you've given yourself. You have gathered your image details along with the way you feel and benefit from acknowledging and developing your process. This process will strengthen your packing efforts. Knowing your Power Colors will also make creating looks easier because your clothing will play well together.

Things needed:
- Your itinerary. Check what the weather will be for that time of year.
- Create a checklist of each daily event. Think through your whole day. Example: If you are going to a conference: (a) the morning is mostly sitting as you listen to a panel of experts, (b) off to lunch with some key people (c) in the afternoon, you are the presenter then (d) dinner with a group at a local casual place outside of the hotel. You will want to dress and pack accordingly for all these different activities during that one day. In your big purse, you might have a different scarf you can add, and a second set of earrings, so you can transitions from your day outfit to a dinner outfit. Add a light wrap for the weather change.
- When packing, always include double duty items like travel boots or shoes that will work with a few outfits so you get the most use out of every item.
- Always bring a great pashmina (wrap) in cotton, wool or cashmere! It is the best double-duty item.

As you choose each outfit lay it on the bed with all the details. Lay each outfit side by side; you may see some overlap, or perhaps see a few items that can be changed but still give you the look you want with fewer items. Tanks, shells, tees and wraps are light and change your look easily. Once everything is laid on your bed, take a photo of it to make packing easier. If you can take a photo with you IN the clothes, that would work too.

For travel that includes business and pleasure:

You'll be creating a wardrobe of crossover items; business and pleasure must be on your mind as you lay items out. A great blazer, worn with a skirt for business, can easily work with jeans and a tee for the next leg of your travels.

Checklist for *Effortless Packing*© with Style

[ ] Itinerary (the one provided or create one if it's a do-it-yourself trip)
[ ] Look up weather typical for the time of year in that location

Important considerations:
Your Audience, Goals, Activities, length of stay, laundry on location

Create a Travel Capsule or Cluster (two different words for the same thing), which includes twelve garments that easily mix and match with each other, avoiding all black!

  [ ] 4 to 6 Tops: shake it up and consider blouses, dressy tees, jersey
       wraps, sweaters etc. Mix prints and solids
  [ ] 3 bottoms: pants, skirt, shorts—depending on your preferences
  [ ] 1 or 2 dresses or skirts—choose those that are easy to layer with a
       blazer or sweater

Accessories: Scarves, statement necklace, bracelets—whatever makes the exclamation mark for your outfit!

  [ ] Shoes: Heels, flats, boots and athletic. What you need will depend
       on your activities.
  [ ] PJ's
  [ ] Undergarments—consider the list or outfits above
  [ ] Bonus item: A wrap or Pashmina in a neutral color such as grey or
       khaki is the perfect item to use as a blanket or pillow as well as for
       drama or warmth.

Most Importantly:
  [ ] Photograph each outfit (with you in the clothes or them laying on a
       bed)

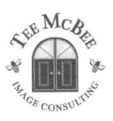

Ask yourself ...

IN THE LAST THIRTY DAYS, WHAT PATTERNS ARE EMERGING?

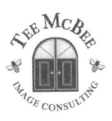

Ask yourself ...

In the last thirty days, are people interacting with me differently?

_____

_____

_____

_____

_____

_____

_____

_____

_____

_____

_____

_____

_____

_____

_____

_____

_____

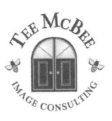

Ask yourself ...

IN THE LAST THIRTY DAYS, WHAT SELF-CARE HABITS HAVE I STARTED?

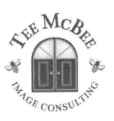

Ask yourself ...

HOW MANY SELF-CARE HABITS AM I STILL DOING?

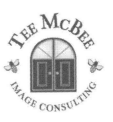

Ask yourself ...

IN THE LAST THIRTY DAYS, AM I GETTING CLOSER TO MY **PERSONAL** GOALS?

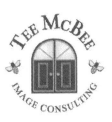

Ask yourself ...

AM I GETTING CLOSER TO MY **CAREER** GOALS?

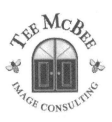

Ask yourself ...

IN THE LAST THIRTY DAYS, AM I EMBRACING MY SUPERPOWERS?

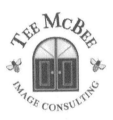

Ask yourself ...

IN WHAT AREAS OF MY LIFE DO I NEED HELP TO ACCOMPLISH MY GOALS?

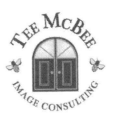

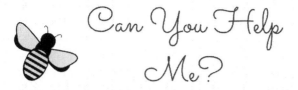

Can You Help Me?

Writing books is a joy. But to get them into the hands of those that need my book is really out of my hands and *squarely in the hands* of my readers.

People read reviews before purchasing so:

Could you please write a review on **Amazon**, **Barnes & Noble**, **GoodReads** or anywhere else you frequent.

It would mean the world to me.
They say if you don't ASK you don't get. :)
Thank you,

Traci